C0-ANG-378

# We Will Be Healed

2017
DF

# We Will Be Healed

*Spiritual Renewal for Healthcare Providers*

Susan J. Bliss

acta
PUBLICATIONS

BV
4910.9
.B557
2006

**We Will Be Healed**
**Spiritual Renewal for Healthcare Providers**
by Susan J. Bliss, RPh, MBA

Edited by Marcia Broucek
Cover Design by Tom A. Wright
Text Design and Typesetting by Patricia A. Lynch

Unless otherwise indicated, scripture quotations are from the *New Revised Standard Version Bible*, copyright © 1989 by the Division of Christian Education of the National Council of the Churches of Christ in the USA. Used by permission.

Scripture quotations marked NIV are taken from the *Holy Bible, New International Version*®. Copyright © 1973, 1978, 1984 International Bible Society. Used by permission of Zondervan. All rights reserved. The "NIV" and "New International Version" trademarks are registered in the United States Patent and Trademark Office by International Bible Society. Use of either trademark requires the permission of International Bible Society.

AUTHOR'S NOTE: Anecdotes in this book are based on fact; however, names and details have been changed to preserve privacy.

Copyright © 2006 by Susan J. Bliss

Published by ACTA Publications, 5559 W. Howard Street, Skokie, IL 60077-2621, (800) 397-2282, www.actapublications.com

All rights reserved. No part of this publication may be reproduced or transmitted in any form or by any means, electronic or mechanical, including photocopying and recording, or by any information storage and retrieval system, without permission from the publisher.

Library of Congress Catalog number: 2006935395

ISBN 10: 0-87946-326-0
ISBN 13: 978-0-87946-326-7

Printed in the United States of America

Year 12 11 10 09 08 07
Printing 8 7 6 5 4 3 2 1

# Contents

**Faith**

For my husband, Joe,
whose patience makes the impossible,
possible.

# INTRODUCTION
## Too Tired to Heal

*"Come to me, all you that are weary and are carrying heavy burdens, and I will give you rest. Take my yoke upon you, and learn from me; for I am gentle and humble in heart, and you will find rest for your souls. For my yoke is easy, and my burden is light."*

—Matthew 11:28-30

The hospital pharmacy phone rang at four-thirty in the afternoon, the Friday before Labor Day. The home-care nurse said with some irritation (which was not like her), "Martha Barnard is being discharged from four-west, and the doctor still hasn't given us orders for pain medications." Martha's kids lived far away, and her adult foster-home caregiver was growing increasingly nervous.

Martha was an eighty-six-year-old woman, withered down to skin and bones at ninety-five pounds. Her fearful blue eyes looked out at the world with early dementia. Sometimes she confused her doctor with her daughter. "Becky, Becky," she'd call, waving her arms, "Don't be late to school." When she had shattered her hip in a fall and it had been surgically repaired, her moaning hadn't stopped for days.

Everyone on the staff—pharmacists, the floor nurse and the home-care nurse—had been calling the attending physician all day. A compassionate woman, the doctor often volunteered at the free health clinic and usually had a quick smile for me when we passed in the halls. She had managed a large patient load for years. When I finally reached her, I said, "Martha Barnard is set to go home, but there are no pain meds on her discharge orders."

"She has enough pain medication at this time," the doctor replied abruptly.

"Martha was on oxycodone 5 mg, every four hours in-house. She'll at least need a tapering dose," I said.

"She has meds at her home," she said and hung up.

The staff was stunned. I verified the orders with the floor nurse, who said the doctor had dropped the orders in front of her, turned and left. I read the orders to Martha's foster-home caregiver and told her to contact the doctor after hours if Martha was in pain.

When I showed the orders to the evening pharmacist, he said, "I'm going to be hearing from the doctor by ten P.M." We all shook our heads, shocked that the physician would let a feeble little patient go home with nothing for pain.

Everyone who works in healthcare, whether seeing patients, preparing medications, billing insurance or working in a lab, has witnessed the burnout of a coworker. Someone who always made the extra effort for people deteriorates to minimal performance. An angry specialist speaks through his answering service, informing the patient that he *never* returns calls on weekends: "Just go to the ER." A hospital nurse says she is "off in five minutes" and claims she doesn't know who wrote the sheet of discharge prescriptions that can't be filled without her help. A pharmacy technician answers a question that requires a pharmacist's knowledge to answer, while the professional on duty continues talking to his broker on the phone.

No matter how many times we hear the same symptoms, determine the same diagnosis or dispense the same medications each day, the moment we stop seeing people as individuals, we risk dehumanizing them and ourselves.

Why do we burn out? Why do we become too tired to heal our patients, too tired to heal ourselves? I believe staff burnout is cumulative and often starts because *most of us have no control over our workload.*

Before a three-day weekend or on the morning after a big medical story breaks on the news, a physician's office may suddenly be expected to care for many more people than usual. The same day, several key support people may call in sick.

A hospital increases its income by ramping up the day-surgery unit to record capacity, and veteran nurses have nightmares about patient safety.

A pharmacy manager is suspended for unprofessional behavior, with no explanation given to the public. Angry, exasperated people complain about the lousy service that the remaining exhausted pharmacist is able to provide the rest of the week, suggesting he is incompetent.

Every day, healthcare workers function at emergency speed, even in routine jobs. The normal workload at most physicians' offices, hospitals and pharmacies is the absolute maximum amount of work that can be done each day, every day. As the waiting room fills up, patients use the extra time to think of more questions to ask their healthcare providers. No matter how healthy patients may be, they can always find one more problem that requires help.

We also become fatigued because *there is no escape from the job.*

Medical professionals often spend their workdays in complete denial of their physical needs, eating "on the run," if at all. In many medical offices the phones are forwarded to the answering service during the lunch hour, while the staff frantically catches up on the morning's patients and paperwork. In some pharmacies the entire staff consumes liquid meals instead of eating solid food.

Healthcare professionals learn to avoid talking about their work socially because inevitably someone will produce a health problem, seeking free advice. Some practitioners become virtual recluses at home, refusing to answer the phone in the evening. Children and spouses of healthcare professionals often grow to resent the incessant beeper and the intrusion of other people's problems that penetrate every private moment at home.

Why would anyone work this way? Why don't we all just turn off the phone and go home on time? Don't other people do that?

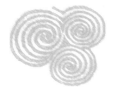

*Caught between the demands of work and our inability to turn patients away, we take on this endless load because we believe we're here to help people.*

Caught between the demands of work and our inability to turn patients away, *we take on this endless load because we believe we're here to help people.* Trained to respond to every person, we take every request seriously. If a question goes unanswered, if the patient with potentially serious symptoms can't be seen today, if the pharmacy runs out of a drug, we have failed. If the emergency room overflows, if the hospital runs out of beds during a pneumonia outbreak, we are still bound to help everyone. We cannot leave any important work until the next day.

Workdays always run into overtime, and we are often called in to cover for colleagues. Dinner may routinely occur at nine P.M. after a day-shift job. If we can stand up and keep food down, we are expected to work our shifts, no matter how we feel. Yet those we see socially are genuinely puzzled that we don't want to volunteer for a good cause in the evening. Don't we want to *help?*

The weight on our shoulders increases with *our patients' limitless desire for good health, and our systems' nearly limitless capability to respond to each request.* Although some health problems are very minor, quality medical care demands that we evaluate each patient carefully. The "worried well" may respond to every physical change as though it were an emergency. When we spend much of our time "healing the healthy," we can feel exhausted without accomplishing much.

The healthy we heal may include the person who demands elaborate vaccinations and prescriptions for travel on the day before she leaves on safari; the impatient person who insists on a last minute appointment and then doesn't show; or the man who intends to live forever and wants a free twenty-minute consult about mega-dose vitamins, despite the nurse's jammed workday.

How can we be merciful to ourselves and still get our professional work accomplished?

In his short ministry, Jesus left us a trail of clues about the mystery of healing, and the difference between mercy and sacrifice. Hounded day and night for his healing touch, the New Testament records that Jesus often slipped away for some peace and privacy, while the crowds incessantly searched for him. Despite many trips through his homeland, he didn't heal every sick person in Israel. It does not seem that was his primary mission. Why do we think it is ours?

Breaking bread one night with a crowd that included the local contingent of tax collectors and other riffraff, Jesus explained his choice of dinner companions: "It is not the healthy who need a doctor, but the sick. But go and learn what this means: 'I desire mercy, not sacrifice'" (Matthew 9:12-13, NIV).

Was Jesus talking about our patients, or us? Just a few years into our health careers, we ruefully come to understand about the sacrifice. But what about the mercy? Must we show mercy to ourselves in order to show it to our patients?

Who will care about the diabetic physician who seldom has time for morning exercise, or the nurse who works a double shift despite her back pain? What happens when the respiratory therapist works overtime on a twelve-hour shift while her sick child waits at daycare? When the lab tech bruises one arm in twenty because the vacuum tubes have been poorly made, does it hurt him to hurt his patient? It seems that it must.

What rest is there for the tired healthcare employee? Who will lift this burden? Who will help all of our patients if we are too tired to care, too tired to heal?

This book is written for those of us who know we don't have all the answers but are asked endlessly by patients, anyway.

It is for those of us who wonder if we should leave healthcare and do something easier.

It is for those of us who feel lousy while we work, who have trouble saying no to every request.

It is for those of us who have a sneaking feeling that it's not all in our hands...no matter what the media, the malpractice insurance suits and the public proclaim.

It is for all of us who labor by day to work with the sick and toss and turn at night, wondering if we have done everything we could and done it right.

My professional field is pharmacy, and I have had the privilege of getting to know patients, professionals, caregivers and health systems in depth. This book was written in snatches of time before and after long workdays, often with sore feet propped up on a chair while scribbling on a tablet. Working in senior centers, pharmacies and the physician's office, attending rounds or checking oceans of bubble packs headed for the nursing home, I am just one of the millions who care for patients every day.

There is help available. Come meet the Master Physician, who knows that the healing arts flourish in partnership and were never intended to be a solo practice. Let his light illuminate the darkness. There is no waiting, there is no cost, and he has an opening—right now.

*Susan J. Bliss, RPh, MBA*
*Hillsboro, Oregon*

# The Endless Load

# The Healing Pool

*"Do you want to be made well?"*
*—John 5:6*

J esus stood near one of the city gates of Jerusalem on one of the Jewish holy days. He had entered the small, stagnant world of the chronically ill who surrounded the pool of Bethesda, which was said to have healing powers. According to legend, an angel would come down and stir the waters, and the first person to enter the water would be healed. Porches surrounded the pool, and dozens of the lame, blind and ill encamped, waiting for a miracle.

Gospel writer John doesn't tell us whether people were actually healed by the water, but those clustered on the porches around the pool believed it. One man in particular had looked for that miracle day after day, centering his life on the cure he expected. Since he had no one to help him, however, he was never able to be the first to slip into the water when it was disturbed. He had lain there, disappointed, for thirty-eight years. The longer he was sick, the more his illness overtook his world. Fixing an unblinking stare at the glassy water, he saw nothing else.

Catching the man's eyes with his own, Jesus asked him, "Do you want to get well?"

Jesus had witnessed the power of belief in overcoming sickness. From his own family life, he may have remembered home remedies his mother had administered, the way her loving touch, even more than the cooling cloth or the herbs she prepared, relaxed him and soothed his fever. He'd also seen people of faith carry the sick to the priest for a blessing, believing that God would respond. And each time a person was healed, they believed more fervently. As an adult, every time he entered a village, the blind, the lame, those weary from caring for the sick met him expectantly, believing his touch would heal them. When the people witnessed a blind man's eyes opened, or a disabled child walking for the first time, people ran to share the news and the crowds grew even larger.

Yet here at Bethesda Jesus did not offer to help the man into the water the next time the surface rippled. Nor did Jesus ask for details about the man's sickness, what he had done all those years to try to help himself. Jesus did not offer to do what the man expected or professed to want.

Instead, Jesus pulled him away from the hope of the healing pool, looked straight at him and asked the simple question, "Do you want to get well?"

Jesus understood that the desire to be well is at the core of healing. Healing requires faith and effort from patients, as well as healthcare providers, and none of us can completely predict the outcome. It requires great courage for patients to explore new treatments or assistance, especially if they suffer from long-standing illness. Disabled people may need to use a motorized wheel chair and learn to use other adaptive aids. Acutely ill people may need to submit to extraordinary surgery, treatments or drugs.

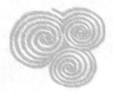

*Professionals and patients may get so caught up in the process of care that they focus on the disease, lab tests and prescriptions instead of the health and wellness the patient still has.*

Professionals and patients may get so caught up in the process of care that they focus on the disease, lab tests and prescriptions instead of the health and wellness the patient still has. Patients may no longer see that they are able to become well; they may see only the battle against their sickness. They may feel like the sum total of the treatments, the pile of empty prescription bottles stuffed into a dresser drawer, and the medical bills accumulating on the kitchen counter.

Illness also isolates patients. After many years of failed attempts at healing, some patients no longer believe they are able to get better. They may be tired of taking advice from others and feeling guilty that they cannot help themselves. Eventually, they may stop asking for help, and it may seem that they no longer *want* to get better. They may see only their *disabilities*, failing to appreciate their *abilities*.

For the man at the pool at Bethesda, the world had shrunk to his disabilities. His only experience was that patio full of misery, staring at the water and waiting for it to stir. Bethesda had become a handicapping support group, confining the sick and drawing all their energy into waiting for a cure.

It must have been shocking to the Son of Man to see this colony of people passively waiting for a miracle, while the Miracle Himself could hardly find time to eat, often working day and night to heal the sick who followed him. Along the roadsides of Judea, the blind, the epileptic, the lepers and those barely able to walk had groped for Jesus' hand, pleading for help. One paralyzed man inspired such friendship and hope in his friends that they tore open the roof above Jesus' head and lowered their friend to him, demanding his attention!

Yet here, clustered on the sunburned porches skirting the pool, people had become so isolated that they apparently hadn't heard about Jesus, much less found a way to intercept him in his travels about the city. The man at Jesus' feet apparently did not recognize him as the healing prophet that others could not stop talking about.

What did Jesus know about the man lying on his mat? Was the man actually capable of walking? Was he paralyzed, or had his limbs atrophied from disuse? Had he abandoned the idea of ever helping himself? In thirty-eight years, had his family or the local physicians offered some kind of help to him that he had refused, insisting instead on waiting for the miracle to occur? Had he ever offered up prayers of gratitude over the years for the fact that he *could* see, hear, think and converse? It seems doubtful that he had ever attempted to help anyone else. He certainly did not say to Jesus, "Lord, there are others more ill than I; help them first." Had others given up on him, after he gave up on himself?

Whatever Jesus knew about him, Jesus understood that this man needed to reclaim his desire to be well. Jesus did not reach over to help him up, but instead commanded, "Get up! Pick up your mat and walk!" (John 5:8, NIV) This man, who had waited for someone to help him all his life, exercised his faith at last and leaped up.

This was not a passive healing. *If the man by the pool had not responded to Jesus' question and subsequent command to get up and try to walk, he would not have been healed.*

It is precisely their desire to be well that enables patients to reach back to us and receive the full benefit of what we can offer. Extending God's healing touch to our patients, we just may be able to stir the waters.

DEAR GOD,

*We recognize that healing is an active process and that those who are ill must want our help for improvement to take place. Help us to be patient for that moment to come, when we are able to extend our very best to the ones who want to get well. Some may not be ready to be healed; some may not listen to what they don't want to hear, or may be angry that we can't lead them to a complete recovery. Help us to forgive them for this, remain ready for the signs that they want our help in the future, and be willing to give again.*

*Help us also to be patient for your part in our work, because all healing comes from you. We are your assistants, and like the sick we must reach to you for help and be willing to receive it in this, our healing art.*

*In Jesus' name,*

AMEN.

# Hearing the Call

*Now there are varieties of gifts, but the same Spirit; and there are varieties of services, but the same Lord; and there are varieties of activities, but it is the same God who activates all of them in everyone. To each is given the manifestation of the Spirit for the common good. To one is given through the Spirit the utterance of wisdom, and to another the utterance of knowledge...to another faith...to another gifts of healing...to another the working of miracles, to another prophecy, to another the discernment of spirits, to another various kinds of tongues, to another the interpretation of tongues. All these are activated by one and the same Spirit, who allots to each one individually just as the Spirit chooses.*

*—1 Corinthians 12:4-11*

*As [Jesus] walked by the Sea of Galilee, he saw two brothers, Simon, who is called Peter, and Andrew his brother, casting a net into the sea—for they were fishermen. And he said to them, "Follow me, and I will make you fish for people." Immediately they left their nets and followed him.*

*—Matthew 4:18-20*

Twenty-five years ago, the United States was gripped by a deep recession. Young and new to the northwest, the only job I could find was field interviewing for a market research firm anchored in a busy shopping mall. My job was to interrupt shoppers and ask them a string of questions about which household products they used. If they "qualified," I would try to convince them to do a more extensive interview that would give my company information and would get the participant a free product, a taste test or a few dollars.

"Do you or anyone in your household currently use the following products? Shaving cream? Deodorant soap? Hemorrhoidal preparations?" I quickly learned to be both direct and polite, keep my voice low, smile, and above all not take rejection personally. On the average, ten "approaches" might net me one person who would do an interview. Since I was paid only for completed interviews, I earned less than minimum wage.

Many interviewees were so surprised when I approached them that they would answer my questions, and I became one of the company's best inter-viewers. I learned to distinguish parents from the childless (parents have spe-cial stress lines in their facial muscles), could guess ages as accurately as any sideshow barker (when you really need a mom between thirty-five and forty to get a paycheck, you get good at this), and was brave enough to recruit bikers, punk rockers or whomever would talk to me.

When I decided to apply to pharmacy school and my friends asked me why, I told them I already knew I could talk to strangers about personal care issues, so I was a natural for pharmacy. Several years later, I walked up the steps of the pharmacy school building for the first time. I was looking for a new career and probably would have laughed to hear it described as a calling. I simply believed in science and in my energy to apply it to helping others.

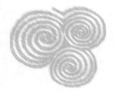 *Those of us who cared the most about our patients were the most frustrated with our jobs. How could we heal the healthcare system itself?*

A few years after I began practice, surprised at the chasm between my pa-tients' real medical needs and the delivery system that restricted their access to care, I became disillusioned with my field. Those of us who cared the most about our patients were the most frustrated with our jobs. How could we heal the healthcare system itself? Some of us became politically active, some worked within professional groups, and some—like me—considered grad school. Over-whelmed with my own lack of power to improve the system, I considered leaving the field entirely. My employer's career assistance program provided counseling, which ironically led me away from that employer and toward graduate school. I was accepted into an MBA program at a Christian college.

My business courses were radically different from pharmacy school, and my professors brought their faith in God into the classroom, which was foreign and strange to a science major like me. New questions came to mind: What is the difference between a job and a calling? Is it possible to earn a living while listening to that call?

I am not the first person who has been surprised by the answer to these questions. Jesus lived the first three decades of his life in a small town, learning his father's trade of carpentry and contributing to his family's support. He attended the local synagogue and lived a faithful life that was so ordinary that it was barely mentioned in the Gospels. One day, it was no longer enough for him just to earn a living. Did he know what was coming? Was he surprised that he was called to leave behind the hammer and saw and employ new tools?

The Old Testament is filled with stories of prophets who were called by God out of an ordinary life to live in a radical new way. Some walked out of obscurity, as Jesus did, and became leaders and prophets of God. Others, like Moses, were called to abandon positions of power and influence and follow God's lead, even through deep valleys of uncertainty that spanned a lifetime. Others were led by God to more subtle missions. No matter where or when they were called, the lives of those who listened to God were never the same.

Eighteen months into my business degree I received my own calling. Shaking my professor's hand the last evening of his wonderful leadership class, I felt something open in me that had been closed for a very long time. I entered a restless period of several days. The feeling built that I must do something; I called my professor and asked if he had time to talk. Even though it was a week before Christmas, he immediately made time to see me.

Despite his intense and demanding professional career, it was his simple, child-like faith in God that struck me most. He said he did not have all the answers, but he had some ideas about where to look. Showing the characteristic humility that I have since found in followers of Christ, he gave me some suggestions for reading and on finding a church, and he prayed with me.

On Christmas Day, I walked into a church. I hadn't worshiped God in twenty-five years, but I had fumbled through a conscious prayer a few times, my weary heart slowly turning toward God.

Turning to look back at my profession, I saw the bleeding need for change within it, the bone-deep fatigue and frustration experienced by nearly every healthcare professional. Having completed the bulk of my graduate degree, I was finally in a position to step out of healthcare. But just as obviously, God was calling me right back into the healthcare mess.

I was determined to find new ways to improve patient care and to also enrich the workday of those around me. Descended from generations of entrepreneurs, I created a business and struggled through plan A, then plan B, and most of the rest of the alphabet. Active in professional organizations, I got to know the leaders in my state and was surprised to find new allies. I wrote about my field, working up to an ethics column in a national pharmacy news magazine. Some of my ideas eventually surfaced in consensus opinions on critical issues. The seeds of this book were germinated during those years, despite tremendous obstacles in my personal life. Still undergoing great change, I now occasionally take a break, look back at where I started, and see a glimpse up ahead of what I might be able to do with God's help.

In the end, being called and the destination of that call may be startlingly different. In healthcare, *it's not the job itself but the way it is done* that matters most. Nearly any set of skills can translate into a healthcare job. Every technological advance, contract or training session can lead toward better patient care, or away from it. The technicians who maintain the HVAC systems in hospitals and clinics, the food service workers who nourish patients and employees, and the administrators, marketing people, printers, drivers and warehouse workers who run patient care systems may all benefit the sick quite directly. Some medical professionals may migrate into public policy jobs, drive change through business creation, or move into research, clinical trials or software writing—all in the hope of working to improve patient care.

There is *profession*, and there is *calling*. They are not necessarily the same. I realized that I could work for the highest-paying and least responsive system I could find, go home and drown my sorrows in excess spending, and complain to my friends at CE meetings...and still be a professional.

My calling, on the other hand, may involve projects that span years, bringing professionals together to start new projects, or writing to motivate those who can effect change. My true life's work may even require changing to a position that allows me the time to pursue that calling, even if it is accomplished without pay in my spare time. For me, the difference between profession and calling is how I feel at the end of the day—and whether I am able to build a better future for the patients in my care.

*Dear Jesus,*

*Guide me to make use of every natural talent I have,
and develop in me the courage to follow your call
for my life and my work. My profession needs deep
commitment and creativity to flourish; the patients
in my care need my investment of thoughtfulness to
develop the system that serves them, as well as the
individual care decisions I provide for them today.
Show me that hearing and yielding to this call will open
up the richest path of patient care and professional
development possible, no matter what limitations I
seem to encounter.*

*In your name,*

*Amen.*

# Too Tired to Heal Myself,
# Too Tired to Heal Anyone Else

*For everything there is a season, and a time for every matter under heaven…*
*a time to break down, and a time to build up…a time to seek, and a time*
*to lose.*

—Ecclesiastes 3:1, 3-6

Jesus lived the years of his life with purpose and patience, finding his unique rhythm as a human being. He apparently knew how to rest and recognized his need for it, even if he wasn't always able to slow down when he needed to. Gospel writers, who wrote with such economy, often mentioned that even the Son of God grew hungry and tired, sought quiet and rest, and was frustrated at times. Starting his ministry in his thirties, Jesus learned to balance the endless needs of others with his reserve of physical energy.

When my own professional career began in my thirties, I quickly found the limits of my energy and had to re-learn how to rest. The people who taught me the practice and satisfaction of deep rest were the Mexicans; I returned to the same quiet stretch of their Pacific coastline dotted with a few tiny towns many times. It took me years to learn to slow down.

That first winter, my husband and I went to Mexico for a week, our first vacation in eight years. We studied a guidebook, wrote ahead to several small hotels, mailed off deposits, bought our tickets, and had no idea what to expect.

The first surprising aspect of rest we learned in Mexico was to *expect the unexpected.*

In both large cities and small towns in Mexico, we were the only ones who regarded our schedule as carved in stone. Miss the bus? "*Mañana,*" someone would say, "there will be another one tomorrow." In a country where paper is scarce, word of mouth replaces written information. At one hotel, we asked for towels after we checked in and three shifts of housekeepers passed the request "*mas toallas*" from one to the next for an entire week, and our shelves overflowed. Mexican Spanish did not translate exactly using my "Spanish" phrase book. Finding a bathroom was an adventure. Food was far better than any Mexican restaurant at home, as we tasted wonderful new ways to enjoy familiar ingredients. Local people celebrated each meal with a flourish, buskers hopped aboard city buses, played guitars and passed the hat, and everyone tolerated crowding with great acceptance and humor.

We then learned to *disconnect from measured time.*

Shops in Mexico mysteriously close for hours during the day, but reopen until late in the evening. "*Un pequeño momento*" (one little moment) to Mexicans is loosely interpreted to mean a half hour, two hours or the next day—not the next line in my date book. People do not attempt to apply makeup, balance the checkbook, or make calls while walking down the street. Time relates to the passing day, not the precise instant.

We learned to *do nothing while at rest.*

This was the most difficult change for me. I had always multitasked my vacation time—reading a book at the poolside, planning every trip downtown with a shopping list of gifts for friends—and ceased action only when asleep. To be conscious and not engaged in any activity was completely foreign to me. Mexican families will eat, laugh, talk and sit at the table in a restaurant for an hour or two. No one brings the check until asked. Women will sit outside watching the kids play in the evening for hours. Hard working and physically tired from manual labor or tending a shop for ten hours a day, people stop trying to accomplish anything when it is time to rest.

I began to *completely separate my play from my work.*

I've watched Mexican dads with their kids leap through the surf for hours, caught up in the joy of the moment, unselfconscious about how they looked. In North America we often contaminate play with our restless pursuit of the ideal equipment, schedule intense lessons to learn how to play, and admire ourselves in our exotic workout gear. Measuring our improvement and applying other efficient work behaviors can make a day off for recreation more work than a paid job.

I learned to *laugh and stop taking my life so seriously.*

Kids everywhere naturally exploit every possible opportunity to have fun and are delighted to involve adults in their jokes. One boy in a small fishing village burst out laughing when I bought a frozen fruit bar at the drug store and began enjoying it, since in Mexico only kids eat them. He laughed every time he saw me for a week! My husband and I took the bus between beach towns frequently; the little bus tipped and lurched down the rutted road as we almost fell over on the kids next to us. Despite their attempts to be polite, when we started laughing, so did they.

When we got on the wrong bus or were caught by a big wave and tossed up on the beach with a swimsuit full of sand, passersby would smile and communicate without words. No matter how we botched our restaurant Spanish, waiters always brought the food with a flourish and served us something that tasted great.

The Mexican people intrinsically understand that we control very little of our lives, and therein lies the delight in our days.

The most difficult part for me to learn? I learned to *rest as much as I need.*

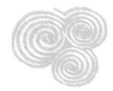

*The most difficult part for me to learn?
I leaned to rest as much as I need.*

Mexicans do not willingly work two full-time jobs apiece, nor would they work late *and* get up early. Sundays, whole families from babies to grandparents find a nice spot on the beach and swim and laugh for hours and hours, until the equatorial sun sinks behind the mountains and everyone is completely tired and ready for dinner. Mexicans don't "squeeze in a quick nap" or hurry to get to their fun destination. They have fun along the way.

We watched people leisurely painting small watercolors, fishing for dinner with nothing more than a hook and a line, or sitting in the town square and giving their full attention to a concert. The moment at hand was the best moment of the day—not an hour from now, but right here and right now.

When planeloads of stressed-out American tourists land in Mexico, they often complain impatiently and charge right out to buy straw hats and beachwear before grabbing dinner and downing a couple of quick drinks in time to watch the sunset. Days later, the same people are so slowed down and relaxed while waiting to fly home that the incoming arrivals spilling out of planes seem to vibrate with tension.

On our first trip to Mexico, my husband and I were desperately tired. When the cabin door of the plane opened, a blast of humid air hit us, and we were swept into an airport bus full of impatient Americans. I couldn't see over the six-footers as we crowded through customs and couldn't understand any of the overhead announcements. Sweat ran into my eyes as we stood in the sun, searching for a bus to get us to our air-conditioned hotel. We dragged our wheeled suitcases five cobblestoned blocks after the last stop and sighed in frustration over the elaborate sign-in procedure at the hotel desk.

On the way home, in contrast, we milled aimlessly around the airport. I peeled our last orange, the juice dripping from my fingers. We still couldn't understand the fuzzy overhead announcements, but we didn't care. The plane was quite late. My husband—tanned, relaxed and looking better than he had in years—laughed: "Maybe it won't come today. Maybe we'll get to stay another day or two!"

I've heard it said that once you go to Mexico, you never quite come all the way home again. A little more of Mexico lingers in me every time I return. I tell people that I'm spending my retirement there, a week or two a year. People ask me when I'll stop going, and I say, "When I finally get it right." I mean get the *rest* right.

I am getting close.

DEAR CREATOR,

*Just as you rested on the seventh day of creation, teach me to value rest. Lead me to deep rest, allowing it to present itself as a vital need that must be satisfied with life-giving time and space.*

*We are not intended to work ourselves to death, no matter what our work may be. No human mission, including that of your Son, has ever been so important that it supersedes the need for rest, play and enjoyment.*

*So be it!*

*In Jesus' name,*

AMEN.

# The Wounded Healer

*For we do not have a high priest who is unable to sympathize with our weaknesses, but we have one who in every respect has been tested as we are, yet without sin.... In the days of his flesh, Jesus offered up prayers and supplications, with loud cries and tears, to the one who was able to save him from death, and he was heard because of his reverent submission. Although he was a Son, he learned obedience through what he suffered; and having been made perfect, he became the source of eternal salvation for all who obey him.*

—Hebrews 4:15; 5:7-8

*"Very truly, I tell you, when you were younger, you used to fasten your own belt and go to wherever you wished. But when you grow old, you will stretch out your hands, and someone else will fasten a belt around you and take you where you do not wish to go."*

—John 21:18

In our careers as healthcare providers, there are days when we feel poorly, but staffing is short and our patients need us, so we do everything we can to be at work and get through the day.

Sometimes an infirmity of our own hits us with particular acuity when we confront a patient with the same illness who is not doing very well. Professionals are loath to share details of their own battles with health. One of the chief unwritten rules is "Don't add to your patient's burden," expressed within the Hippocratic oath as "Do no harm." We are trained to set the patient's needs before our own, even at the expense of our own comfort or rest.

Taught, administered and regulated by imperfect human beings, all medical professions observe this deep, unwritten paradox: The professional most able to understand illness is the one who has experienced it; yet sometimes the job requires us to suppress, even ignore, our own infirmities.

Few would disagree that Jesus was a compassionate and insightful healer. With human hands and no formal medical training, he was able to heal those he encountered and even empowered his human companions to do the same. There was at least one moment in his ministry when the crowd became so excited about his powers that they tried to forcibly make him king. They may have thought his dramatic healings were the first sign of his sovereign ascent.

Yet none of Jesus' healing miracles spoke to his human companions as deeply as the evidence of his triumph over mortality, written in the scars on his body. Even his most loyal followers did not understand his divine yet human nature until they encountered him alive that first Easter morning, still bearing the scars of his ordeal.

Weeks after the resurrection, Jesus appeared again to his disciples, this time waiting for them on the shore of Galilee while they were out fishing—unsuccessfully. When Jesus' words caused a miraculous catch of fish, his friend Peter leapt from the boat and swam to him, recognizing that it was Jesus.

As Jesus handed Peter some of the fish he had cooked for breakfast, Peter could see the healed scars on his arms. It was the scars that proved Jesus to be both man, capable of suffering, and also God, capable of healing. The scars, the evidence of his new, eternal life, were necessary for Peter and the others to believe and accept his help to heal their own wounds.

The book of Hebrews makes a scholarly case that Christ's suffering was a tool in God's hands, enabling him to fully understand and experience the very depths of human life, including pain and death. When we look at Christ the healer, we can see his power, his confidence, his certainty. Yet his daily pain of being misunderstood, the rejection from the very people he tried to heal, and his battle with those who would end his ministry before it started more accurately characterize his healing days here on earth. If we look at Jesus and disregard his scars, we miss the point of his life. Despite his perfect expression of faith in God, it is his experience of human life, with all its pain and suffering, that makes him like us and leads us toward eternal life.

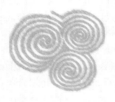

*If we look at Jesus and disregard his scars, we miss the point of his life. Despite his perfect expression of faith in God, it is his experience of human life, with all its pain and suffering, that makes him like us and leads us toward eternal life.*

Henri Nouwen, the French priest and writer, thoughtfully explored and defined the concept of the wounded healer in his book of the same name. A writer of great simplicity yet one so profound that his work requires meditation and time to understand, Nouwen said that neither aloofness nor wallowing in our own pain is the best way to reach and assist others. The imperfect experience of Jesus' life shows us how our own difficulties can enable us to help our patients.

Nouwen wrote, "When the imitation of Christ does not mean to live a life like Christ but to live your life as authentically as Christ lived his, then there are many ways and forms in which [to] be a Christian."

The point of surviving suffering is not the suffering itself, but to enter and understand the suffering of those around us. We do not need to experience every pain and every illness in order to have empathy with others who suffer, but we do need a willingness to allow our own experiences and lives to become a touchstone, where we can meet others and reach out to them.

As do many of my patients, I experience migraines, an invisible, annoying and long-lasting form of pain. I can usually manage the pain of a migraine and finish the day, unless a patient stops and talks endlessly about how much her headache hurts and how much time she has to take off from work for it. Then I begin to feel sorry for myself.

At the end of one very long day at the pharmacy, a woman in her mid-forties stood in line to pick up her migraine prescription. The surge of patients abated, and I said to her, "I get migraines too. What do you do to prevent them?"

She described how she and her doctor had weeded through the causes of her headaches, using both prevention and treatment strategies. Then she smiled at me and said, "One time, I had this terrible migraine. I tried everything. Nothing worked at all. I'm a Christian, so I opened my Bible, laid my head down on it, and it finally went away."

The next week at work, a migraine began boiling under my temples. Since I can't take sedatives or pain drugs at work (and virtually nothing works for me anyway), I silently asked Jesus for some help with this one. 'Please help me get through the day,' I thought, ignoring for a moment the ear-splitting din of ringing phones, the line of muttering patients, and my short-handed staff working furiously. Within a few minutes, my forehead was not as warm and the pain had eased away.

I remembered the face of the woman who had talked to me the week before, and I thanked the Wounded Healer, who had worked through her, for helping me.

DEAR JESUS,

*Your extraordinary life, your experience of work, of suffering, of healing, of joy, was lived in the most ordinary of surroundings. It is through your human life attuned to God that I, too, am able to reach God.*

*Let me be grateful for the opportunity to open myself to those I care for, allowing them space and time to express their needs. Let me make use of my own infirmities to reach out to them with empathy.*

*Help me to remember that you needed to care for your body and soul within your human life, just as I do. Allow me to recognize and accept the help you offer me through others, as you offer them help through me.*

*In your name,*

AMEN.

# Mercy

*"Those who are well have no need of a physician, but those who are sick. Go and learn what this means, 'I desire mercy, not sacrifice.' For I have come to call not the righteous but sinners."*

—*Matthew 9:12-13*

One day, Jesus walked by the tax collection booth near his home and noticed a man sitting there, busy at the task of keeping his accounts. Jesus stopped to talk, and before he walked away he said to the man, "Follow me." Matthew closed up shop and followed Jesus the rest of the day, intrigued enough to invite him to dinner later at his home.

Whatever Matthew's religious practices, he must have been quite skilled at extracting tax from the community, and his dinner companions would most likely have been other tax collectors. Seeing Jesus and such riffraff elbow to elbow, the Pharisees were alarmed and pulled Jesus' disciples aside to ask, "Why does your teacher eat with sinners?"

Hearing this, Jesus turned to the Pharisees. Matthew must have looked intently at his guest, probably expecting Jesus to open a discussion of sin or perhaps suggest a ritual offering that would please God and the Pharisees, since in the legalistic framework of ancient Jewish life, atonement for sin always involved the sacrifice of animals.

Instead, Jesus said told them it was not healthy people who needed a physician, but the sick. He quoted Hosea, saying, "But go and learn what this means: 'I desire mercy, not sacrifice.'" Jesus' call to "mercy, not sacrifice" is a profound call for those of us serving the public. Like Matthew, some of us have become distanced from those we are supposed to serve, reducing them to accounts to manage and charts to file.

I was once working for a large pharmacy that cared for the chronically disabled, and my employer had contracted to care for Jessica, an eighteen-month-old child whose drug profile was filled with anti-seizure medications and neurological drugs. Every drug-refill request for Jessica required the whole day to battle through the insurance system. Every contact with her physician's answering service resulted in a call back from a different doctor or a pager number for the resident on call.

Jessica lived in the custody of her aunt and uncle. After talking with them several times, it became clear to me that our delivery service was the main reason the family used our pharmacy. One morning, after our chief pharmacist had spent the night calling her physician and running medication out to her home, he groaned, "We have to do something about this." We were all exhausted with the aunt's calls, dreading the sound of her voice on the phone.

I began investigating. In a year of care, we'd run emergency refills out to her house at least twice a month. The guardians couldn't read well, so they didn't call for refills until the medication packages were empty. Of the three physicians at the neurology clinic, two of them begged off on taking care of Jessica; her family had exhausted them with their needless panic. The last woman physician I got on the phone said, "I don't have time to take care of this child! I could spend the entire day on her alone, and I have dozens of other patients."

"I don't have time, either," I said. What were we going to do?

I voiced my concerns to the chief pharmacist: "The family can't understand her medications, and we are doing emergency management for this child. We're hanging ourselves out to dry, liability-wise. The parents need to find a closer pharmacy or take responsibility for picking up her medications themselves."

The chief looked at me. "I've been thinking about this for a long time, too, and I agree with you. Will you take care of this?"

When I reached the agency nurse at Jessica's home, I summarized our predicament: "This kid has a different doctor for every problem. I can't get them to spend five minutes with me on the phone. The parents don't seem to understand what's going on. Tell me about her."

The nurse sketched out Jessica's medical problems for me. Jessica had been born prematurely at thirty weeks. She had neurological deficits and mood instability consistent with fetal alcohol syndrome. When I looked at the picture of her clipped to her files, I could see she had the clear facial markings of fetal alcohol syndrome.

Jessica had been in and out of the hospital three times in a year for re-evaluation. Thin and drastically underweight, she required sophisticated care every time she was dehydrated from a childhood illness. But her guardians could not distinguish true emergencies from routine needs, and they regularly used the ER for non-emergencies. In addition, her erratic home care contributed to repeated hospitalizations, a higher risk of critical seizures, and constant pressure from her insurance carrier. Jessica simply was not getting what she needed; it cost her family, it cost the healthcare system, but it especially cost her.

After some persistence, I reached Jessica's case manager. She agreed to set up a monthly review of her medications, medical care and home status. When the beleaguered physician finally returned my call, we discussed the clinical merits of the drugs being used and designed simpler treatment for her. When I called Jessica's aunt, I said "We will be delivering new prescriptions tonight. Stop giving her the old ones."

"God bless you," she said sincerely. I was taken aback. Jessica had become merely an irritation to me, a frustration. I had never met her. I had been storming around for two days, trying to resolve this impossible problem, and now her aunt had blessed me.

Somewhere between the endless phone calls and the struggle to care for her, Jessica almost slipped from being a human being in our care to just another annoying problem on the other end of the phone line. Worn down from trying to fit a seriously ill eighteen-month-old's pharmaceutical needs into our cost-controlled system, we had become remote bureaucrats, accomplished at papering over our feelings with impatience, rolling our eyes as we groaned, "Oh, not *this* again."

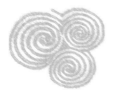

*In the tail-chasing sacrifice of our hours and energy, we had forgotten that it was our mercy she needed most. She needed someone to watch, to gather up her story, and to demand that it be listened to.*

The drugs, the medical treatments, the deliveries were not the point. *The point was to care for this child of God, a little girl who did not choose to be ill.* In the tail-chasing sacrifice of our hours and energy, we had forgotten that it was our mercy she needed most. She needed someone to watch, to gather up her story, and to demand that it be listened to. She needed our mercy, my mercy. My part was to bring us together so all we could look at the needs of the child—not my needs, her family's needs, her physicians' needs, or the needs of the accountants in the healthcare system.

Sitting down to dinner alone at nine-thirty that evening, I thought long and hard about the difference between mercy and sacrifice. My throbbing feet finally at rest, I reflected on Matthew's long-ago meal with Jesus. Just like my colleagues and me, Matthew was a contractual thinker, a logical man who knew every line of the law. Some time after that dinnertime conversation, he left his tax ledgers behind to become one of the twelve disciples, empowered to drive out evil and heal every disease and sickness. The man who had once reduced his profession to prying every piece of gold from the fists of his neighbors, now took up his mission to freely share God's grace. Healing others with the power given him, he trusted that God would provide food and shelter and that people would receive him in the name of the One who had sent him.

I thought about my own profession—pushed by cost containment, eternal staffing shortages, and delivery limitations. The needs of every patient compete with the mountains of work for everybody else. As the speed and volume of work grows, we are tempted to see patients as problems and caring as an unnecessary expense.

Jessica's medical care had nearly become an afterthought, and caring for our own needs had also been nearly forgotten. Physically fatigued from a workload that could double on any given day, our compassion wore down as our tired legs pounded back and forth on cement floors. Was it really necessary to sacrifice our own health to work in healthcare?

Was there mercy for me or for Jessica?

I realized that right about then, Jessica's aunt would be giving her the bedtime dose of her new medication. It may have taken extra time to resolve the child's drug treatment, but the doses would now be easier to give, fewer times each day, and the monthly case review I had insisted upon would save all of her healthcare providers many hours every month.

Putting up my feet, I picked up a cookie and examined it carefully, as if it contained a secret. What if I took a break every afternoon, no matter how busy the day, and showed myself a little mercy for ten minutes? What might I be able to do for another patient like Jessica, with a little less sacrifice and a little more mercy?

*Holy One,*

*We learn to be merciful by first experiencing your mercy. In a world gone mad with greed and grown cold with indifference, it's too easy to view the lives and needs of those around us as mere accounts. Without showing mercy to ourselves and those for whom we are bound to care, we can all be sacrificed to the clumsy structure of our institutions, sometimes completely eliminating the "care" within our medical care systems.*

*Remind us that Jesus first cared about those he healed and then worked to free them from their infirmities. His mercy, his deep regard for the patient, was the heart of his care for the sick and the reason why those in need still call his name without hesitation, knowing he will hear and respond.*

*Finally, work through my professional skills, inspiring me to remember the point of all I do, translating your love for me through my actions on behalf of the patients in my care.*

*In Jesus' name,*

*AMEN.*

# Decisions

# Discernment

*Now they had been sent from the Pharisees. They asked him, "Why then are you baptizing if you are neither the Messiah, nor Elijah, nor the prophet?"*

*John answered them, "I baptize with water. Among you stands one whom you do not know, the one who is coming after me; I am not worthy to untie the thong of his sandal."*

*The next day he saw Jesus coming toward him and declared, "Here is the Lamb of God who takes away the sin of the world.... I myself did not know him, but the one who sent me to baptize with water said to me, 'He on whom you see the Spirit descend and remain is the one who baptizes with the Holy Spirit.' "*

—*John 1:24-27, 29, 33*

What should I do?

One bitter December night, I sat cross-legged on my bed, my best reference book opened to a page of warnings about a sedative drug. Christmas music drifted softly from my radio as pellets of ice chattered down the windows. It was Christmas week, and I was on call for two thousand nursing-home patients. My pharmacy license barely three weeks old, I had answered a page and received my first scary prescription order. My gut instinct told me not to dispense it.

The order was written for a patient in a residential facility that did not have the trained personnel and equipment to maintain life support. But the "black box" warnings in my reference book emphasized the necessity for full life-support backup when administering this drug. When I called an area hospital for more information, the seasoned pharmacist on the other end of the line said, "Don't dispense it! Seven patients in this city have died on that drug. I wouldn't have anything to do with it, if I were you."

When I phoned my boss, who had worked in hospitals for years, he told me he knew little about the drug.

"The hospital pharmacist and my reference both say full life-support is vital to using the drug safely," I told him. "Seven patients in the city have died in the last year."

He thought about it for a moment and said, "Go ahead and dispense it. The doctor knows what he's doing."

The pressure on me was tremendous that dark night. How could I make a good decision? How could I disagree with my boss? What if I dispensed the drug and the patient died in a facility that was not safety-rated for the procedure?

In the end, I called the nursing home and told them I would not dispense the drug. About an hour later, the stuff hit the fan.

I sweated through the next twenty-four hours, fielding angry phone calls from nurses at the facility, the physician, and my boss. Everyone's anger seemed aimed directly at me. I was holding things up! How could I insinuate that the physician was not competent?

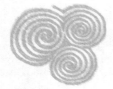

*The rest of us must appreciate that there will be moments of brilliant clarity in our God-given missions, and other days when we will anxiously ask, "Is this the way?"*

When we as professionals make important decisions, we may face the loneliest moments of our careers. The professional license hangs silently on the wall while a colleague waits on the phone or the patient looks to us for a decision. Time seems to stand still, yet there is a moment when we must act. How can we be ready to make a good decision, every time?

Jesus was the only human being who could discern God's path for his life with every breath, every day. The rest of us must appreciate that there will be moments of brilliant clarity in our God-given missions, and other days when we will anxiously ask, "Is this the way?" Whether we are deciding how to help a patient, in what direction to develop our careers, or how to allocate limited resources, we continually need to ask for and listen to God's voice to find our purpose.

Religious writers use the term "discernment" to describe this waiting on God for direction. We can learn much about discernment from the rugged life of John the Baptist. John experienced both times of clear, unmistakable direction from God and times of anxious wondering what his purpose really was.

We don't know much about John's life before his river ministry. He and Jesus were cousins who, though born just a few months apart within a relatively small geographic area, had apparently never met. We also know that John lived in the wilderness, where he was called by God to begin his intense mission.

John was the last of the Old Testament-style prophets: abrasive, fearless and persistent. He lived far from the temple's splendor, preaching and teaching from the waters of the Jordan River to crowds who felt compelled to listen. John looked and behaved strangely, his life stripped down to wearing homespun clothing, foraging for locusts and honey, and following God's plan for his life. There was nothing to distract John from hearing God's call: no family, no possessions, and no power. In the serenity and simplicity of his wild hermitage, he knew his mission exactly and carried it out without hesitation.

From the banks of the Jordan, John preached the Kingdom of heaven. John knew with absolute certainty that God had sent him to break new ground, to instigate baptism, which would turn a generation toward the one who would baptize with the Holy Spirit. He called people to repent, and when they confessed their sin, their separation from God, he washed them in the waters of the river.

John spoke of sharing possessions with those who had none, of working honestly for fair wages, of turning away from extortion and selfish practices, words that resonated later in the teachings of Jesus. When asked if he was the Messiah, John spoke of his mission of preparation.

John had waited and listened for his call, and was ready when it came. One day under the broiling desert sun, Jesus came to the river to hear John. Even though they had never met, John immediately knew that the Spirit of God was within Jesus. When Jesus was moved to ask John for baptism, as hundreds of others had done before, John was instantly ready to follow, and exclaimed, "I am the one who needs to be baptized by you!"

As John witnessed the infusion of the Holy Spirit in Jesus, John's own mission shifted from leading to serving. In one moment, God's Son was anointed and sent on his mission, and John's greater mission ended. John didn't hesitate to offer his support, and even his followers, to this Son of God.

John was later imprisoned by rulers who were afraid of his influence and ability to move people. Far from the wild beauty of the desert, John's action-filled life was reduced to dark days of confinement and physical stagnation, and he struggled to understand the ascending arc of Jesus' mission. Fearful and uncertain of the future, he sent his messengers to ask Jesus, "Are you the one we have waited for?"

Ultimately, John may never have known the true extent of his mission. Yet Jesus later called him Elijah, who had returned to herald the coming of a new age.

I take great comfort in John's life. John shows me that it is possible for an imperfect human being to perfectly discern God's plan for his or her life and to carry out responsibilities with utter faith. During his solitary desert sojourn, John had prepared many years for his short mission.

Creating moments of solitude can prepare us as well to discern the still, small voice of God whispering within us. Sometimes the voice is strong and clear, and our response is vivid and full of action. Other times we must come to the river over and over, trusting baptismal water to wash away our doubt and knowing that God will patiently murmur to us, as many times as we need to hear, the best direction for our lives.

I know that the richness and clarity of my professional decisions improves when I practice quiet meditation and prayer each morning. The practice of listening and being receptive gives God the space to move within me and gives me the time to listen to God's direction. Allowing God's peace to fill me at the beginning of each day makes it possible to find that peace later, in a busy moment. When I return to this peace, I allow God's hand to direct me toward the best decisions for patient care and for my career.

HOLY IMMORTAL ONE,

*Help me grow in my ability to discern your direction
in my life. As I read your word, help me relax in your
soothing presence so I can make decisions in your light.*

*Teach me to wait patiently for your direction. I trust
you to help me make decisions that will be considerate
of everyone involved. Help me to place those affected
by each decision, instead of myself, at the center of my
meditation.*

*Finally, allow me to better understand Jesus' example
of discernment within every Gospel story I read. Show
me that his leadership is truly living water to those of us
who thirst for direction.*

*In Jesus' name,*

AMEN.

# Failure

*He left that place and came to his hometown, and his disciples followed him. On the Sabbath he began to teach in the synagogue, and many who heard him were astounded. They said, 'Where did this man get all this? What is this wisdom that has been given to him? What deeds of power are being done by his hands! Is not this the carpenter, the son of Mary...? And they took offense at him.*

*Then Jesus said to them, "Prophets are not without honor, except in their hometown, and among their own kind, and in their house." And he could do no deed of power there, except that he laid his hands on a few sick people and cured them. And he was amazed at their unbelief.*

*—Mark 6:1-6*

*All in the synagogue were filled with rage. They got up, drove him out of the town, and led him to the brow of the hill on which their town was built, so that they might hurl him off the cliff. But he passed through the midst of them and went on his way.*

*—Luke 4:28-30*

There is a cold and lonely moment when it becomes clear it's all over. The accumulated good will, the good intentions are used up. All that's ahead is failure.

In the life of any project, relationship or career, there are crisp, defining moments that separate failure from success. Listeners either get excited about the message and invest themselves in it, or they walk away. The one who attempts to kindle a friendship is either welcomed or ignored. A career gathers energy and success or it slips backward.

In the medical arena, great new ideas in patient care rise up from professionals in daily practice—from imaginative researchers, floor nurses or administrators, any of whom may see new possibilities in the large institutions they serve. Every healthcare professional worth his or her training has had a new idea to improve the job or take better care of patients. Some are modest proposals, new ideas to streamline the work process. Other projects span years of preparation and rely on the investment of faith and seed money to get started.

These new ideas must then be brought before the Board of Directors, the Chief of Staff or the Administration for consideration. Those of us who propose the ideas swallow hard and wait for our leaders to make their decisions. As if listening for the wind, we watch and wait for a reaction. Sometimes, it's a bone-chilling blast that feels like failure.

At one of those defining moments, feeling renewed and invigorated, the Son of God traveled toward his hometown of Nazareth. He'd left home months before, coming to a critical commitment after wandering in the desert for weeks. During his months of travel, his eyes must have filled with delight as the touch of his hands and his bold calling out to God brought wholeness to sick people. Did he smile at their amazement? Did he cry tears of joy with them when they grasped the true source of his power?

By the time Jesus returned to Nazareth, he had healed many, while demonstrating the love of God in the ordinary, imperfect lives of men, women and children. Surely everyone had heard of his miracle of turning water into wine at the famous wedding in Cana. Surely people in nearby villages had heard about subsequent miracles of healing—sight regained, pain removed, walking restored. Surely people in his home town had heard of these things.

On the road to Nazareth, Jesus' human heart must have filled with the expectation of a happy homecoming. Maybe he anticipated helping the chronically ill he'd known all his life. Although the New Testament is mysteriously silent about the years during which Jesus grew up and worked in Nazareth, Jesus must have seen people suffer: the blind beggar who depended on townspeople for food; the arthritic widow who could barely drag a water jug home from the well.

Mark's Gospel tells us that Jesus was in Nazareth for a few days, just before the Sabbath. But his homecoming was not greeted with celebration. Few of his neighbors placed their faith in this man they'd known since boyhood. There were no mighty miracles, no examples of blind faith, no dead raised from their funeral processions. Instead of cries of "Hosanna!" or "Be merciful to me, Son of God!" echoing through the streets, the mood of the townspeople was subdued.

When Jesus read from the scripture on the Sabbath, the people became incensed at his confident claim that he was the Messiah. Their lack of faith must have jolted him, because Mark writes that Jesus "was amazed at their unbelief."

In a chilling portent of Good Friday, his own people, those who should have been happiest to hear this good news from a native son, turned on him. His words stirred doubt, then anger, then cries of "Blasphemy!" Jesus could have been killed then and there by the furious mob. Somehow, he managed to escape, inexplicably unrecognized.

One more scene probably happened that day. Down the road, after fleeing the angry mob, Jesus probably sat down to catch his breath. In the scuffle the dust must have stirred, making his feet dusty. Off came the sandals. Did he slap them together, knocking off the dust of Nazareth, leaving it behind forever? There is no record that he ever returned. Few miracles were performed in Nazareth, and even the dust from the streets was probably unwelcome to his tired feet.

Later, Jesus incorporated this metaphor into his directions to the twelve when he empowered them to heal and forgive and sent them off to surrounding towns. He told them to carry no money, to accept the hospitality people gave them, and to neither curse nor dwell in the towns that rebuked them but to shake the dust of those streets from their sandals and go on.

Maybe these are Jesus' best directions regarding failure: just move on. Shed whatever threatens to stick to you as a reminder of that place, and move on. There are thousands more miles to travel. Heal others. Move on—to the next patient, the next job, the next town, if need be.

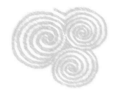

*Maybe these are Jesus' best directions regarding failure: just move on. Shed whatever threatens to stick to you as a reminder of that place, and move on.*

It's sobering to realize that Jesus met failure and rejection again and again. Even as some people rushed to him and clung to him for comfort and healing, others doubted and plotted against him. Jesus' human heart must have been wounded by the disbelief of those who threw his words back in his face. Ultimately, he witnessed the unspooling of his organization and the seeming failure of his mission. As he faced the misery, humiliation and abandonment of the cross, Jesus felt the sting of self-doubt and fear that comes with the prospect of failure. Yet he did not succumb. His perfect faith in the One who sent him enabled him to complete his unique mission.

Everyone who works within healthcare will experience failure. It is inevitable. Disease lingers. Patients die. Inspired projects meet an untimely demise, sacrificed to inexplicable budget cuts that seem to target the experimental, the creative, and the most needed new programs while attempting to apply first aid to the rest of the system as it wails from its own limitations.

To remain in healthcare—despite multiplying responsibilities, huge workloads, and seemingly endless demands from patients—we need to rise above our failures. We need to listen carefully for those who ask for and appreciate the help we can give. Most of all, we need to approach every patient and every project with confidence, knowing that Christ has been there before us, and works along side us, every day.

*Dear Jesus,*

*No matter how many times my projects fail, help me to recall your example of steady faith in action. Just as in your life, it may take me a long time to harvest the first fruits from my work. There may be many tough days, many failures on the way to success.*

*Remind me that you enable me to die to this life of failure and disappointment and to rise again with you in resurrection, every day of my life. Because of your ultimate devotion and faith, your failure and death become new beginnings for me.*

*In your name,*

*Amen.*

# The Healing Spirit

*When he saw the crowds, he had compassion for them, because they were harassed and helpless, like sheep without a shepherd. Then he said to his disciples, "The harvest is plentiful, but the laborers are few; therefore ask the Lord of the harvest to send out laborers into his harvest."*

*Then Jesus summoned his twelve disciples and gave them authority over unclean spirits, to cast them out, and to cure every disease and every sickness.... These twelve Jesus sent out with the following instructions: "...as you go, proclaim the good news, the kingdom of heaven has come near. Cure the sick, raise the dead, cleanse the lepers, cast out demons. You received without payment; give without payment."*

—Matthew 9:36-38; 10:1, 5, 8

April comes at the end of the long season of lifelessness and turbulent weather in the northern United States. As the first shoots of spring bulbs push up from the death of winter, plants that were well nourished the year before swell toward the spring sun and bloom. But plants that starved in fall droughts are often too exhausted to grow, putting out futile buds that quickly bloom, consume the plant's store of nutrients, and suddenly wither.

So it is with the sick, who often struggle through the winter, only to fade just before the warm weather and die.

A few years ago, I worked in a demanding geriatric program that served those in the last few years of their lives. The staff geriatricians were raised in cultures that revered the aged and built strong faith communities. MD's, nurse practitioners, RN's, pharmacists, and a host of other professionals, social workers, aides, and support personnel worked closely in teams to keep our frail population in community care.

My pharmacist friend Sandy and I often worked late, took our beepers home and innovated our way through the drug formulary, the capitation budget, and the insolvable health problems of our patient population. One day we blew up *two* microwaves trying to compound special suppositories that relieved one patient's nausea. At Christmas, we survived a desperate siege of the flu to get to work and care for our patients. All through the winter, the patients were very sick, but we felt barely able to care for them.

Cuts in insurance coverage had forced exhausted administrators to reduce hours and increase the workload, so we never seemed to have enough help, time or resources. Many jobs seemed to involve moving stacks of paper or screens of data from here to there, leaving workers uncertain about what they were accomplishing. Many of us wondered why we did this for a living. The exuberance we had felt at the start of our careers seemed to flicker at the end of winter, just before the season slipped into spring.

In April, one of our stable, long-term patients spontaneously decompensated, and her mood disturbance resurfaced in eruptions of dissociation. She spiked wild fevers, suffered seizures, and boomeranged wildly out of control. Her geriatrician frantically changed her medications every day and sat by her hospital bed every evening. When she died, he was exhausted as well.

Sandy and I turned to each other and wondered, how could there be a God who would allow such misery to overtake both patients and those who helped them?

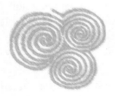 *As Jesus shared his skills with his disciples and taught them to heal, he provided a model for the development of the healing spirit.*

What it must have been like for Christ to travel on foot to dozens of small villages, working alone at first, without help and without a home? As he taught, healed, and offered God's forgiveness, he naturally drew followers. Months after he began, perhaps he reached his human limits and spent a night in prayer. The next day, he began to choose his assistants, building and training the team he needed to help him.

The disciples were by no means perfect. They watched, squabbled, and often fell behind. Yet long before the fires of Pentecost anointed them with the Holy Spirit, Jesus gave them the *authority* to heal the sick, raise the dead, and drive out evil spirits (what would probably be understood as psychiatry or neurology today). As Jesus shared his skills with his disciples and taught them to heal, he provided a model for the development of the healing spirit.

*The healing spirit requires acknowledgment that no one can do it all alone.* As word of Jesus' healing touch rapidly circulated throughout Judea, he had to face the finite amount of his human energy. Even the Son of God recognized the need for help, and he selected a dozen people to help him.

*The healing spirit means that to serve increasing numbers of patients some of the work must be delegated to others.* Early in his mission, Jesus demonstrated that no human being could personally extend this healing touch to every person in Israel, let alone the rest of the world. This is still true today: All healthcare does not have to be carried out by physicians.

*The healing spirit requires leadership and inspiration.* Jesus' ability to ignite the healing spirit, even in the unskilled, is a model for medical recruitment, training and retention. The healing spirit requires continuous investment in leadership and the training of new practitioners, so that all healthcare workers can see the purpose of their work and know that there will be enough hands to get the work done, now and in the future.

*The healing spirit thrives when leaders develop work teams, sharpen the skills of assistants, monitor their progress, and provide help when needed.* Jesus later sent out seventy-two assistants, working in teams, with detailed instructions about how to work, where to work and how to respond to rejection and refusal. As his organization grew, he set them up to work independently, advancing his work and message and preparing the way for his return.

*Nurturing the healing spirit requires recognition and reward.* Gospel writers were sparing in their accounts, but at least once they recorded Christ's exultation when those he had trained and sent out into the world returned with stories of miracles from their own hands. Jesus often told his followers that they would not be forgotten; by extending God's caring into the world, rewards would come their way. Jesus himself was astonished that so few stopped to thank him for healing—a clear sign that every human heart and even the heart of God listens for a sign of appreciation for the work of healing. Every leader and every healthcare system needs to remember and recognize the good work done every day by healthcare workers.

*The healing spirit recognizes that we cannot heal every patient.* The disciples were not able to heal every patient they saw; some were referred to the Master Physician himself. We, too, may benefit from a colleague's assistance. When additional skills are needed, it is important to refer patients to others who can help.

*The healing spirit is a true partnership with God.* After the disciples' exuberant return from their healing mission, Jesus reminded them of the true source of their healing power. When we remember that it is our dedication, not our achievements, that God loves the most, we will stay grounded in humility and gratitude.

*The healing spirit requires regular rest, refreshment and rejuvenation.* Christ himself worked within the limitations of a human life. When he grew tired, he stopped to rest, eat and socialize. He also spent quiet time alone in communion with God. He was philosophical about these limitations, remarking that "you always have the poor with you" (Matthew 26:11). Each of us participates in God's larger plan when we know when to rest and when to find additional help.

*The healing spirit requires us to recognize our limits.* The only human being who could heal himself is Jesus Christ. Lifting himself from his own grave, Jesus is the only human being in history to overcome this finite lifetime. Every other being on this planet, including those trained in the healing arts, will need help to cope with his or her own illnesses and limitations. Fortunately, Christ is always available to help.

GRACIOUS GOD,

*You have invested us with the heart, the mind, and the ability to learn how to help others heal. Through us you extend the wonders of health science and its service to other people. Help us to recognize and treasure this healing spirit within our colleagues and ourselves.*

*Remind us that we are your assistants in this work. True healing is a mysterious combination of your intervention, the intrinsic capabilities you designed within the human body, and our care and training. We may not always understand our role in healthcare, but we know you will warmly reward our efforts when we fully participate with humility and dedication.*

*Thank you for this, our work, and its unique satisfaction.*

*In Jesus' name,*

AMEN.

# Letting Go

*As he entered a village, ten lepers approached him. Keeping their distance, they called out, saying, "Jesus, Master, have mercy on us!"*

*When he saw them, he said to them, "Go and show yourselves to the priests." And as they went, they were made clean.*

*Then one of them, when he saw that he was healed, turned back, praising God with a loud voice. He prostrated himself at Jesus' feet and thanked him. And he was a Samaritan.*

*Then Jesus asked, "Were not ten made clean? But the other nine, where are they?"*

—*Luke 17:12-17, NIV*

Jeff was a little boy who lived on our street for part of a year. Previously, he and his mom had lived in a dilapidated old house with a dozen people, until she became pregnant again. Jeff's aunt and uncle had convinced them to move in with their family, a few doors down from our house.

My husband and I were amazed at the courage and generosity of our neighbors and the way they lived their faith, trying to protect the unborn child and help the sister get back on track again. The whole family attempted to deal with the situation as best they could, but Jeff was kind of forgotten. Impulsive, whiny and sad much of the time, Jeff had trouble concentrating, was underweight and wheezy, and had a wistful, lost facial expression. His learning disabilities and asthma made me wonder what he'd been exposed to as an infant.

Jeff shuffled around the neighborhood in his hand-me-downs, hands jammed in his pockets, watching the other kids whiz by on their bikes. Though other families on our street did not have a lot of money, most of the kids got a new bike every couple of years, and they were quite proud of having the latest color, gleaming handgrips and the perfect size.

Crowded out of garages, bikes were left on the sidewalks or in the front yards of most homes, and Jeff learned to ride by bumming them—swiping them, really. He was small for his age, and we'd see him pumping hard, a twenty-four-inch kid on a twenty-six-inch bike. Usually he'd put the bike back in the right yard, but sometimes the kid who owned the bike would catch him, make him get off after a squabble, and then ride by him at top speed, rubbing it in. Jeff hardly had a toy to his name, let alone a bike, and he was already seven years old.

Jeff loved to talk to my husband, Joe, while he was watching Joe repair the car, set up the ladder and clean the gutters, or mow the grass. A good-hearted kid, Jeff offered to help do chores around the yard. He ached for attention. One spring Saturday, we did one of our morning "bike clinics" for the neighbor kids, when we'd shine up our own bikes and share the chrome polish, the oil can, and the paint cleaner with all comers. Jeff lurked in the background, just wishing.

"That kid needs a bike," my husband said to me. "Why don't we get him one?" Our own budget was tight at that time, but a few blocks away lived a man who collected old bikes, donating them or selling them to kids who really needed them for a small price. "Let's see if we can find Jeff one," Joe said with a grin.

Joe bought a good used bike from the man and collected parts to repair it. Wheeling it out the next day, he asked if Jeff could come over and help clean it up. Other kids congregated in curiosity as the two of them began to work on the bike. Jeff helped Joe put new extra-tough tires on the rims, shine the chrome and prepare the fenders for painting. The bike was exactly Jeff's size. "What color do you think it should be?" Joe asked him. I bought rustproof paint in green, Jeff's favorite color, along with new handgrips and reflectors.

The next day when the paint was dry, they put on the new seat and installed the reflectors and handgrips. When it was done, Joe asked Jeff, "How does it look?"

Then Joe pulled up the kickstand and handed it to Jeff. "This is your bike now; thanks for helping me shine it up."

That little kid's face twisted in an unbelieving expression, his eyes bugging out. Then he kind of panicked, grabbed the bike and raced off on it. Freedom! He rode his new bike until dark, his mom calling and calling him for dinner. The smile on his face, the shock that someone would just give him something he needed has lingered in my mind all these years.

Months later, Jeff's little brother was born. Skinny and sad, the baby looked like his big brother and had the same plaintive, screechy cry. The little family moved away in a few months, refusing more help from their relatives.

Looking back at that spring, I see that the hard part of giving is to give in an open-handed way—and then to let go.

I am reminded of the way Jesus gave the gift of healing freely. He healed all who asked him for help. He made no effort to exert control over the person's future, except to encourage each one to praise God. Some may well have gone right out and re-injured the same limb or contracted another disease. Some probably did things that were foolish, dangerous, or even hurtful with their newly healed body.

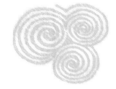

*Jesus healed all who asked him for help. He made no effort to exert control over the person's future, except to encourage each one to praise God.*

Our professional experience in healthcare opens us to the realities—and limits—of healing. We know that some patients may do the exact opposite of what we prescribe. Some need many tries to quit problem drinking, for example. Some who have worked hard to level off diabetes will begin to ignore diet, medications and exercise. Some may not be able to afford good follow-up care or medications, or their medical problems may be a direct result of abuse, poverty, malnutrition, or a host of other ills that we can do nothing about. We know that very few will *fully* comply with treatment and many will boomerang back to the ER or the medical office only when the symptoms worsen—sometimes too late for us to make a difference.

In many of the healing narratives in the Gospels, we see clues that Jesus felt the same frustration and disappointment in helping the sick that we do. More than once, Jesus walked away from the crowds who sought his help, to rest and refocus his attention away from their endless demands. His healthcare "career" spanned just two or three years, but during that short career, he showed signs of fatigue with the public's lack of appreciation and lack of trust. God's own

Son must have sat down after an exhausting day sometimes, head in his hands, and wondered, 'Why don't they get it? Why don't they get me?'

I think Jesus knows exactly how a doctor feels the day he or she loses the fight to save a life and the family unleashes their wrath. God knows patients unload all their troubles on the most compassionate of nurses, then go out and do exactly the things they are told they should not do. He knows all the lab tests in the world will not make up for the patient who continues to make terrible choices and there is no drug that will cure selfishness or mean-spiritedness. He knows healing people is far more complicated than removing symptoms.

Yet Jesus continued to heal without judgment. Our healing commitment must also be free of judgment about whether or not a patient "deserves" our care. To treat patients fairly and consistently, we must separate the things we can do to help them physically or emotionally from the circumstances in which they find themselves. We care for those in jail. We reach out to kids whose parents feed them poorly or who rarely have a good night's sleep. We clean up accidents, no matter whose fault, and offer emergency care to all comers, even though some will walk out of the ER as soon as they can stand and go right back to doing whatever got them admitted in the first place.

That long ago summer, Jeff moved out of the neighborhood a few weeks after he rode away on his shiny green bike, and we never saw him again. Our part in helping others heal may be as small as providing a bike for a forgotten child or as critical as providing life-changing treatment for a patient who is seriously ill. No matter what others need, our part is to give freely, open our hands and heart, and let go.

The rest is up to God.

*FAITHFUL HEALER,*

*Help me to do everything I can to help the patients in my care, knowing that you are the author of all healing. Help me to let go of my expectations, to heal and help freely without judgment about why they became ill or about what they will do next, giving them the same compassion and open-handedness that Jesus provided long ago and still provides today. Help me to transmit the healing that comes only from you, and in so doing I will be blessed to participate in your healing miracles, small and large, every workday.*

*In Jesus' name,*

*AMEN.*

# An Evening at the Improv:
# Comedy and the Health Sciences

*The wise man has eyes in his head,*
    *while the fool walks in the darkness;*
*but I came to realize*
    *that the same fate overtakes them both.*
*Then I thought in my heart,*
*'The fate of the fool will overtake me also.*
    *What then do I gain by being wise?'*
*I said in my heart,*
    *'This too is meaningless.'*
*For the wise man, like the fool, will not be*
    *long remembered;*
*in days to come both will be forgotten.*
*Like the fool, the wise man too must die!*
                        —Ecclesiastes 2:14-16, NIV

One cold winter night, twenty of us packed into a beat-up high-school classroom, waiting for our first comedy improvisation class to begin. We chatted nervously until the teacher walked in at five minutes to seven. She set up a video camera on a tripod, passed out a questionnaire, and we began. Here were my answers to her questions:

**Why do you want to take an improvisation class?**
*To feel more confident speaking in front of groups, to better handle emergencies.*

**What kind of theatrical experience do you have?**
*High school musical, twenty years ago.*

**What other drama classes have you taken?**
*Never taken one before.*

Before I could chicken out, our teacher set us up with our first improv game. The object was to create a commercial for a new food product while thinking on our feet. We made a circle with the chairs and took turns jumping up in front of the classroom audience, making fools of ourselves. My role quickly went from being the note-taker in the front row of the schoolroom to being the troublemaker in the back. There was so little time to think, the jokes popped right out of me.

That winter, I had become completely frustrated with the long hours of my job. After work, I often caromed into the school parking lot and bolted up the stairs to the improv class after consuming nothing but a hard-boiled egg and a box of juice on the way. I arrived exhausted, but moments into the first theater game I was so absorbed and sweaty from concentration that I forgot all about fatigue and sailed away with everyone else to the land of comedy.

Doing live improv is a lot like being in a scramble golf tournament: Everyone has a good shot now and then. With just a few seconds to respond to a joke, stark—and sometimes Freudian things—fly out and form a sort of Rorschach inkblot of the mental landscape.

'Who are these other people?' I wondered, as we flocked to the vending machines during breaks. I found out that in our group of twenty were a pathologist, a dietician, several counselors, a nurse, and me, the pharmacist. The very best amateur at improv was a physical therapist. I still have her wonderful physical improvisation piece on tape.

Why had so many healthcare professionals come to this class?

Nearly every one of us medical "class clowns" mentioned excessive work stress as a motivation. Even our instructor told us that she began the class because she had been having a difficult year and needed to "do something."

On that simple stage in that old high-school classroom, we each came to a new understanding of ourselves. Here I was, embarrassing myself in front of a group of strangers and enjoying it thoroughly, as the fatigue dropped away like scales from my eyes. The comments that flew out of my mouth showed me how bored I was with my job, how ready I was to take risks. I loved responding to what happened around me and using my wits as well as my feet to make the scene happen. Making jokes taught me that, as Ecclesiastes said, *"The wise man, like the fool, will not be long remembered."* In other words, it's okay to make mistakes and try again.

The prophet Ecclesiastes wandered the philosophical desert for years and often wrote like the prototype of the fire-and-brimstone preacher. In other passages of his remarkable book, he wrote with eloquence about living with wisdom. As a teacher, Ecclesiastes probably summoned his audience, said outrageous things to get a reaction, and then contradicted himself later to evoke the opposite emotion in his listeners. Like a good comedy improv player, Ecclesiastes touched the nerves of his audience, built up anxiety and anticipation, and thus focused attention on the heart of his message.

Jesus, like Ecclesiastes, often said things that nettled people and evoked swift reactions. Other times he taught in a more thoughtful, Socratic style, expecting the listener to walk out into the light of understanding by himself or herself. Jesus was also a gifted storyteller. He captured the details of his rural life with the heart of an artist, filling his parables with personalities familiar to every man and woman who paused to listen. He was a master at improvisation, staging common scenes from everyday life to illustrate his message, handling interruptions and hecklers with great presence. Although the Bible records very few of his funnier asides, the Jesus who cried must have also laughed.

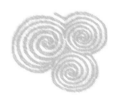

*Although the Bible records very few*
*of his funnier asides, the Jesus who cried*
*must have also laughed.*

Jesus took his message on the road. He never knew just how people would react, except that someone nearly always pointed out the irony of a carpenter talking theology, an uneducated man explaining God to a nation. Yet he tirelessly helped people mend their tattered lives, and I'm sure his days sometimes extended long into the night, just as ours can do.

At day's end, we need to remember that Jesus thought well on his feet, as tired as they must have been.

At the time I took the improv class, I was dancing on the edge of a thin blade, precariously trying to balance my life. Both my husband and I were working for the future, but neither of us was enjoying the present. Creating comedy on the spot with a group of strangers drew me out of myself and reminded me how fleeting our lives are. I felt freer to experiment, and the direction of my work life began subtly to change. I found out that I was an adept improviser. I will never be as skilled as the standouts in that class, but I came to see that if I could laugh at myself my average day would be far easier and I would be more available to those whom I serve.

In a leadership role years later, I needed to train the staff quickly on a serious issue. The staff expected a heavy-handed class, but I surprised them with a comedy skit. They instantly tuned in. The wise man, like the fool, will not be long remembered, but no one soon forgets what they enjoyed learning—including me.

*Dear Jesus,*

*Life has much more comedy in it than I might have once thought. You were a master at handling crowds; you know how difficult it is to get through the day and still be able to laugh. Let me learn from your personal, story-telling style and get over the days I really bomb. Help me to keep my tears and my laughs in balance and remember that you always hold me in lightness and love.*

*In your name,*

*AMEN.*

# As You Give, So Shall You Receive

*"For I was hungry and you gave me food, I was thirsty and you gave me something to drink, I was a stranger and you welcomed me, I was naked and you gave me clothing, I was sick and you took care of me, I was in prison and you visited me."*

*... "Lord, when was it that we saw you hungry and gave you food, or thirsty and gave you something to drink? And when was it that we saw you a stranger and welcomed you, or naked and gave you clothing? And when was it that we saw you sick or in prison and visited you?"*

*... "Truly I tell you, just as you did it to one of the least of these who are members of my family, you did it to me."*

—Matthew 25:35-40

My uncle was a thoracic surgeon, beloved in our small hometown and jolly in personality. Some of my earliest holiday memories revolve around Christmas mornings at his house. One of my cousins called him "Uncle Ho-Ho," since he always passed out the gifts. One year, I had a red felt Santa hat made for him, with *Uncle Ho-Ho* written on the trim with glue and glitter. He slipped the hat on and hammed it up for us. Midmorning, though, he was called in to the hospital for an emergency surgery. When he returned, he said everything went fine except that the patient's family kept staring at his head. The nurses said the family had seen some red glitter in his silver hair and asked them, "Sure he's up to this today?"

For all who enter the health professions, it is understood that holiday duty will be shared among all coworkers; those who don't work Christmas Day will work Christmas Eve. There are three shifts on Christmas Day in the hospitals, three at the nursing homes and three at the ERs, and someone from every department must take call for all those patients.

People who work office jobs rarely miss a holiday event, but they expect the ER, the hospital and the pharmacy to be open when they are sick on holidays—which we are. The confluence of flu season, year-end-deductible fever, and patients' anxieties about spending holidays with difficult family members swell the usual workload. Patients' fears of pain and loneliness intensify. The more fragile the patient, the more they worry about what might happen, calling the ER or the physician's answering service more often.

On Christmas Eve, the candlelight service is usually long over by the time the pharmacy staff finishes the rush of new orders for patients, providing enough IVs and antibiotics to last an extra few days. When I work Christmas Eve, I usually fall asleep on the living room couch very late, listening to Patrick Stewart read "A Christmas Carol" and dreaming about having the week off.

The first Christmas I was licensed, I was the junior pharmacist on the team at a long-term care pharmacy, and I got call for the entire week. After each ten-hour day of work, I drove home and stared at the beeper, waiting for it to fire off. Saturday we had an ice storm. The pharmacy was thirty *long* miles from my house, and the freeway hills were covered with cars spinning out right and left, but I made it in. Then I was trapped at the pharmacy processing a huge number of orders, with only a refrigerator full of the "ghosts of lunches past" for company.

I haggled with two old, deaf sisters who ran the taxi service in a faraway county, trying desperately to get medication to a patient who was fading fast. I played "let's make a deal" with a tired and crabby hospital pharmacist for life-saving drugs. By Sunday I was exhausted. My husband chained up his van and helped me deliver ceftriaxone and morphine myself, since the taxi company was running hours behind. Two days after Christmas, my call ended, and I slept fourteen hours straight as the ice melted.

Medical staff, nurses, pharmacists, lab techs, and all the others who keep healthcare facilities open, form work teams that often function like families. Sharing life and death every day, coworkers understand the intensity of our work lives in ways even our families can't.

The holiday crew may have to cope with a horrible workday, but sometimes the facility can be eerily, almost magically quiet. Footsteps may echo down usually busy hallways, and the sound retreats as silent snow accumulates outside. Late at night, somewhere in the huge building, a patient may die, his or her spirit slipping away into God's waiting arms, freed from a body too tired to continue. In the still moments, it may be just possible to catch the sound of God's heart beating faithfully, encouraging those few working to share a little love and care with one another. In another wing, in the deep dark quiet, a baby may be born, the total focus of some family's attention, much as another child captivated his worried father as he was delivered by his young mother on that first Christmas so long ago.

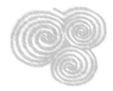

*In the still moments, it may be just possible to catch the sound of God's heart beating faithfully, encouraging those few working to share a little love and care with one another.*

If we believe Jesus when he says, "Whatever you did for one of the least of these...you did for me," and if we believe that we are called to healthcare service—which means caring for other people's loved ones while ours must be alone at home—then I believe our understanding of heaven must expand. Heaven must be a place where all healthcare workers can join their families, friends and coworkers and celebrate Christmas at a ski resort, a beach, or at least around a cozy fireplace. We will have grand and glorious tales about our holidays to share around a holiday feast, instead of another lonely dinner at the hospital cafeteria.

Heaven must be a place where the family we left behind (or never had), the marriage that dissolved while we cared for other people's husbands and wives, and the children who waited up late and still fell asleep before we got home—all will be reunited, restored and repaired. There will be abundant friends and family, and time for all of us to enjoy each other, at holiday time and every day.

And heaven must certainly be a place where those of us who face the demanding families of ER patients or listen to the last-minute panicky calls from those who didn't, or couldn't, plan ahead for the holiday will finally find rest and comfort ourselves. We will sit down in peace. Groceries will be delivered to our home. Dinner will be on time. There will be no more cold plates of leftovers or tired sandwiches from the vending machine. We will sit down with our family and look up to hear thanks from the One whom we served all those holy days at work.

DEAR JESUS,

Let us remember that as we do for one in need,
we do for you; and as we give up and miss out on
family moments now to care for others' families,
you will reward us accordingly in your eternal
Kingdom.

Remind us that the patient who is ill on a holiday
shares in the loneliness and isolation we also
feel, that those who are alone in a hospital room
or watching over a sick family member miss the
familiar tastes and rituals of the holiday as much
as we do.

Pray for us, that we might connect with patients
and coworkers on holiday workdays and find
moments of meaning and peace with each other,
wherever we may be.

And finally, remind us that the holiness of the day
is in our reverence and your blessing; it has less to
do with the specific day and more to do with our
recognition of the rest you provide, whenever and
wherever that rest may come.

In your name,

AMEN.

# THORNS

# There, But for the Grace of God

*"A man was going down from Jerusalem to Jericho, and fell into the hands of robbers, who stripped him, beat him, and went away, leaving him half dead. Now by chance a priest was going down that road; and when he saw him, he passed by on the other side. So likewise a Levite, when he came to the place and saw him, passed by on the other side. But a Samaritan while traveling came near him; and when he saw him, he was moved with pity. He went to him and bandaged his wounds, having poured oil and wine on them. Then he put him on his own animal, brought him to an inn, and took care of him. The next day he took out two denarii, gave them to the innkeeper, and said, 'Take care of him; and when I come back, I will repay you whatever more you spend.'*

*"Which of these three, do you think was a neighbor to the man who fell into the hands of the robbers?"*

*He said, "The one who showed him mercy."*

*"Go and do likewise."*

—*Luke 10:30-37*

One evening, I sank into my recliner after a long day at the pharmacy, put my feet up, and switched on the news. A reporter began a feature about a local homeless shelter. A familiar face popped into the screen. *Carol?* I hadn't seen her in years, but it was definitely Carol. Incredulously, I listened to the reporter ask how she had come to the shelter; she said she no longer had a home.

Carol and I had once worked together at a difficult and low-paying job, retouching photographs for a large studio. She had socialized with many of us who worked there and had been to many of our homes. At that time, she had just moved to the city and was looking for something to do besides go home to dinner with her mother.

The TV still on in the background, I phoned one of our mutual friends. "Carol's in the homeless shelter!" Within an hour, I had rallied our old coworkers and breathlessly called the station to track down the reporter. To protect confidentiality, she wouldn't tell me where Carol was, but she promised to get a message to her: All three of us had room to spare and extra places at the table; we could group together and help her; we were ready.

We waited all day for a call, with no response.

I couldn't believe Carol wouldn't call, and I phoned the station again the next day. The reporter confirmed that Carol had received the message. The reporter agreed to leave another.

We waited another day. I called the reporter back. The response was now clear: Carol knew we had called but did not want to contact us. We never heard from her again.

Why wouldn't Carol call her friends for help? Why had she gone to a homeless shelter in the first place? Although our work relationships had been casual, we had worked hard together in an intense job. At the time, many of us were grateful to earn minimum wage, just enough to buy some groceries. Others, including Carol, worked just to get out of the house. Several of us from that job still contact one another at Christmastime, remembering it as one of the most difficult yet memorable jobs we ever had.

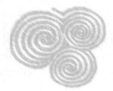

*When we reach out to others, it's important to understand that we may be just one link in a chain. Someone else may be the one whom the person in need is finally able to turn to.*

The TV reporter said that people sometimes get too embarrassed to ask for help. Maybe that's why Carol was in the shelter. None of us could imagine why anyone would check into a shelter before calling every friend she had first. Maybe Carol had never known a friend in such dire straits and assumed that we wouldn't know what to do about it, either.

At times, any of us may be too proud to ask for help, or we may just be tired of asking without receiving. When I remember Carol's face on television that night, it's hard to forget that I will never know what happened to her. I remind myself that even after she turned her old friends away twice, perhaps the next time someone offered help she may have accepted. When we reach out to others, it's important to understand that we may be just one link in a chain. Someone else may be the one whom the person in need is finally able to turn to.

Jesus knew this, walking down the dusty roads of Judea. When he spoke, he knew that on the fringe of the group there may have been those who ached to believe his words but hesitated. Perhaps they needed to hear him several times, or meet those whom he had healed, before they could take the risk themselves. Or perhaps they would one day see Jesus' compassion in the eyes of one his followers, on some other dusty road.

While the New Testament records many stories of healing, there must have been other stories of those who hesitated to ask for help and were not healed. When a leper lying in the street called to Jesus, "Son of God, have mercy on me," another person nearby, perhaps disappointed many times by people who could not help him, must have doubted that this prophet could help him. Though some, such as Nicodemus, were willing to risk their position to have a conversation with Jesus, others may have been too afraid to admit their need and stayed away. When a paralyzed man was lowered through the roof by his friends, landing right at Jesus' feet, another disabled man in the same village may well have refused when his own friends or family offered to take him to Christ for healing.

When Jesus said, "You always have the poor with you," he spoke not only about poverty but about limitation: There will always be more people in need than we can help. The poor in spirit may even include those who are too poor in self-esteem to ask for help, even when greatly needed.

I think of the times in my pharmacy practice when I have gone home worrying about people I would never see again, people who refused the help I offered. The man with the puffy, yellowing face who said he had kidney failure but was looking for an herbal remedy and waved off my plea to see his physician and get back to treatment immediately. The parents with the sick, stressed-out baby with recurrent diarrhea and chronic infections who insisted on going to work while leaving the sick child at the babysitter's. The logger with the blackened, third-degree burn who'd worked for two days after the injury, insisting, "It don't hurt none!" when I tried to chase him into the ER.

All of us who work in healthcare have been haunted by the faces of those who insisted they didn't need our help. What happened to them? Did some other professional or family member finally get the message home? Did a patient's deaf ears finally comprehend that the situation was serious?

Never knowing what happens to those in our temporary care may be the toughest part of caring for patients. Yet accepting people with open arms and releasing them if they're not ready may be the healthiest expression of our caring—and one of the most difficult things about the job.

No matter what we think is needed, our patients will not follow through with any treatment unless they have *decided* to participate. It's their decision, not ours. Our job is not to *take* control but to *place* control in their hands and wait to be asked for help with the healing.

DEAR JESUS,

*Help us to see people as you see them, accepting those who don't want our help while remaining open to those who do. Sometimes we must be the messengers who alert patients about their needs yet allow them to walk away. Just as you did not let your pride be hurt by those who did not ask, help us release the patients who are not ready to accept our help. Give us the grace to let patients make up their own minds, and lead them back to our healing hands in the future when they are committed to receiving help.*

*Just as you were able to hear the broken-hearted and dying who called to you, help us to better hear the calling of those who welcome our help today.*

*In your name,*

AMEN.

# The Thorn in the Flesh:
# When the Healer Is in Pain

*Therefore, to keep me from being too elated, a thorn was given me in the flesh, a messenger of Satan to torment me.... I appealed to the Lord about this, that it would leave me, but he said to me "My grace is sufficient for you, for power is made perfect in weakness."*

—*2 Corinthians 12:7*

*For now we see in a mirror, dimly, but then we will see face to face. Now I know only in part; then I will know fully, even as I have been fully known.*

—*1 Corinthians 13:12*

"This is what I call the 'fainting couch' position." My physical therapist, Jim, had draped me sideways over his knee, the fingers of one hand dug into the inflamed intercostals on my side while I stretched back until the pain released, for a long count of sixty seconds. It was a good thing they put those curtains up between the work benches in physical therapy, because we must have looked ridiculous.

Midway through pharmacy school, I had a two-month case of the flu. When my flu symptoms dragged on, my doctor first thought I had post-viral fatigue. Later, he diagnosed arthritis and muscle inflammation. Even though I was in pain, pharmacy students and licensed professionals are expected not to take any prescription medication for pain while working. I also couldn't reduce my class load without losing a whole year of school. Fortunately, the school health service had excellent and affordable physical therapy services. Jim treated me three times a week for six months, which provided enough relief for me to finish my classroom work by the end of the school year.

After finishing school, I tried hard to find a desk job but wound up working on my feet eight to ten hours a day. Pain traveled up my legs to my neck and shoulders, and I was so tired that I lay on the floor at home during the hours I wasn't working.

I did everything I could to keep my body as strong and relaxed as possible, from swimming several times a week to sleeping adequately to eating well. I learned to use visualization and meditation to distance myself from pain. My husband helped me with stretching and strengthening exercises.

Now and then, I'd stop by and talk with Jim. Once he said, "After a while, people stop talking about the pain so much. I can never decide—do they get better or do they just get used to it?"

I think we get used to it.

Support groups helped at first, but after I had assimilated every practical treatment and philosophy and invented some of my own, I stopped going. Spending my free time hearing people talk about how lousy they felt eventually became a burden, not a help. Most of the patients I have helped over the years—whether they had arthritis, depression, diabetes, or another chronic illness—have had a similar experience. A year of active participation in a support group usually led to a good adjustment to the illness and the acquisition of the skill to manage the symptoms. It's a fine line between adjusting and spending too much precious time and energy fighting a battle you can't win. It's too easy to miss out on whatever good things you can still enjoy—and there are always things we can enjoy, even during pain or illness.

Arthritis is a great teacher. Arthritis taught me that we can be in pain and still be in love. We can be in pain and be happy. The pain can coexist, side by side, with the rest of our lives, and it does not have to be the only sensation we notice. This is the only life we are given. If pain comes as part of the package, we can't stop the pain without stopping everything else too. Over time, we can tease apart the good times and the bad, and make the best of every good moment we receive.

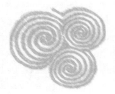

*We can be in pain and be happy.*
*The pain can coexist, side by side,*
*with the rest of our lives, and it does*
*not have to be the only sensation we notice.*

When I allowed Christ to teach me, I learned to appreciate his pain during his life among us. I am sure there were times when he was hungry and tired, when he and his group scavenged from fields for a makeshift meal or simply did without. He obviously ached with compassion even when mortally wounded. Witness his attitude toward Pilate, toward the women of Jerusalem who followed him to the cross, even toward the thieves who died on the same executioner's grounds. Whether the bruises were physical or emotional, Jesus felt tenderness for those in need.

Scripture tells us that Jesus "took our infirmities and bore our diseases" (Matthew 8:17). Did Jesus physically absorb and experience the suffering and pain of every person he healed? I believe he did. In my years of working alongside other healthcare professionals, I have seen that the person who has directly experienced a particular pain—or the miserable treatment for an illness—is often the one most able to understand what the patient needs. Superb training, sheer intellect, and vast clinical study do not orient the professional to the patient's true world of hurt nearly as well as experiencing the same thing. My deepest disappointment in a colleague occurs when a healthy professional arrogantly views a patient's experience not only as foreign but also as isolated or even self-generated.

In the second book of Corinthians, the missionary Paul describes having a "thorn in the flesh." No matter what we think of Paul, or what his thorn might have been, coexisting with this imperfection moderated his arrogant self-determination and deeply influenced his missionary career. The effect of this suffering was positive and profound, and its experience was not wasted on Paul.

The impact of pain was not wasted in my own life, either. A great percentage of the patients I help have chronic pain. My experience enables me to creatively advise them on new ways to moderate their pain, and the smile of relief and appreciation I often later receive is a big pain reliever to me. I now laugh about my aches and know that I have something in common with many, many people every day.

More than a decade has passed since I was diagnosed with arthritis, and I have almost completely escaped chronic pain. Much of the time I am pain free. But sometimes the aching returns when I push too hard for a few weeks or suddenly change my workload. This really is my thorn in the flesh, a dormant reminder that this body is not yet eternal, that this earthly life is anchored to a physical body that needs rest, care and kindness to serve me well.

DEAR JESUS,

*I can learn many lessons through my own pain and suffering. Help me to learn patience and empathy, which will enhance my attitude toward and treatment of the sick. Remind me of my mortality to prevent the sneaking belief that somehow I am the one making healing miracles happen. Help me to recognize the many people who quietly endure physical discomforts and illnesses that are invisible to others. Help me to help myself, to avoid feeling sorry for myself and to do everything possible to ensure that the time I spend with patients is productive and positive for us both.*

*Finally, Jesus, thank you that I can look forward to a day when all of your children are freed from pain and suffering and I can take your wounded but healed hands in my own with joy.*

*In your name,*

AMEN.

# The Kingdom Belongs to These

*People were bringing little children to [Jesus] in order that he might touch them; and the disciples spoke sternly to them. But when Jesus saw this, he was indignant and said to them, "Let the little children come to me; do not stop them; for it is to such as these that the kingdom of God belongs. Truly I tell you, whoever does not receive the kingdom of God as a little child will never enter it." And he took them up in his arms, laid his hands on them, and blessed them.*

—Mark 10:13-16

A child, sick with fever, lies in the arms of her worried father. His face is bronzed and weather-beaten from years of working in the fields from sunup to sundown. He is paid his daily wage according to how much work he does, by the bunch or the bushel, as long as the fruit is ripe and his back is strong. Today it is raining and there is no work, so he makes his way through the streets. He has heard that the healer is in town. He reaches the building he recognizes (he can't read and has no phone), and his worried face sags. Look at the crowd gathered here, all of them seeking help.

The story of the tired father could be straight from the New Testament, but small dramas like this one still take place today. Underneath the surface in our own rich country, beneath freeway overpasses filled with cars, in back of the shopping centers filled with goods, far from winding neighborhoods filled with comfortable homes, another country and economy exists. Tired wage-earners put in sixty or seventy hours each week, washing dishes or sweeping floors and working two or three part-time jobs. Single mothers carry the endless load of parent, wage-earner and caregiver. Homeless families move from shelter to shelter or live in their cars, looking for day labor.

When the kids of these families are sick, the obstacles to care may be nearly insurmountable. They may have to pack up the whole family just to see the doctor. On a hot summer Sunday, a family waits patiently all afternoon at the emergency room, then streams into the grocery-store pharmacy, kids trailing behind the grocery cart. Sick babe in arms, the mother gives a prescription for a costly antibiotic to the pharmacist. The pharmacist calls the ER to haggle for a less costly drug. While on the phone, he watches the family dig through their pockets, counting change and crumpled bills.

The mother weighs the cost of a jug of milk or a package of hamburger against the cost of the medicine, and looks up with faith that somehow it will be enough. She will not leave without finding something that will help her sick baby. The radiant smile the family gives the pharmacist who helps the child is a touch of grace, if he is able to receive it.

These angels unawares often appear to us when we are most burned out on the job. An exhausted office staff, hoping to be home for dinner for the first time all week, receives a father who is even more exhausted. As the man slaps the cement dust off his hands, he overhears a staff member muttering about the time.

"I wish my workday was only eight hours long," he says flatly.

The ensuing silence charges the air, and the staff rallies with a little energy. "What can we do to help?" asks one of them.

It's hard to remember that each patient is an individual when illness seems to follow such predictable patterns. Three weeks into each new school year, the first colds are passed around and the sore throats and ear infections bloom like pesky dandelions. In the dead of winter, and especially in poor economic times, the flu seems to saturate the public with fear, whether they are sick or not. Angry parents may compete for their children's care, especially under the weight of their own frazzled schedules. When the weather clears and the air heats up, the office is filled with injured children, their summer ruined.

It is hard not to respond with compassion to a little person covered in hives, bawling with pain, or suffering from a chronic illness. When the patient cannot speak or explain what is wrong, we must reach back to the very reasons we entered healthcare, to rekindle the flame of our compassion, and *to find some way to help*.

This kind of caring extends to the profoundly disabled, the developmentally disabled, or those with severe psychiatric illness. Many of those who need us the most are unable to articulate their needs or even thank us when we help. The hours spent on the phone with government agencies, insurance companies, and caregivers are worth it when we lock up and go home, knowing that a severely disabled person will stop refluxing all night once he receives the right drug. The only thanks we may receive from a psychiatric patient who finally connects with her trusted doctor may be the blessed silence of the phone, but sometimes that's enough. The bone-deep fatigue of our days lifts a little on the way home, knowing that, today, we made a difference to someone who had no one else to ask.

In the stories about Jesus' healings, often it was the parents of a sick child who were most motivated to seek him out. Traveling great distances, they plodded ahead until they caught up with Jesus, who was also tired at day's end. His disciples often thought he shouldn't be bothered. Perhaps they saw the lines on his face etch more deeply every day as he walked miles in the desert sun, healing those who ran out to meet him at the fringe of each village. But they also saw his tired face soften into compassion. Touching the children lovingly, he told the parents—and his disciples—that this child-like faith was exactly what his new kingdom would require.

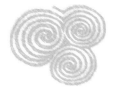

*No matter what he was doing, or how tired he was, Jesus responded with special immediacy when he was presented with the urgent needs of a child.*

No matter what he was doing, or how tired he was, Jesus responded with special immediacy when he was presented with the urgent needs of a child. He once halted a funeral procession and lifted a widow's only son from death, in a spellbinding scene before a huge crowd of mourners. Another day, still filled with the glory of God from his blinding transfiguration on the mountain, this Son of Man heard the single voice of a beleaguered father among the crowd waiting for him on the foothills. The pleading man said his son had writhed in seizures so severe he had been injured many times, while the man could only watch helplessly. Jesus healed the boy of his seizures, teaching his disciples about the power of prayer as he did so.

To Jesus, every child was not only precious but deserved special consideration. Children cannot be expected to know what they need, but they surely need extra care from healthcare providers. Their parents may be exhausted from struggling with their own problems and may not even speak English or understand the language of medical care. Some parents may be disinterested or even hostile, incapable or absent, leaving a child with someone who may not know what that child needs.

If the parent does not explain, we must ask. If something does not seem right, if the examination does not provide answers, if the treatment does not seem to work, we may need to rely on the same intuitive skills that Jesus employed when taking care of children. Every word and every silence, every tear that slips down a reddened cheek may hint at the cause of suffering. For no matter what the state of health of a small child, such suffering is not of the child's doing—or if it is their doing, it is not of their understanding.

Treating pain and illness in those who are incapable of speaking for themselves is one of the gifts of the healthcare profession, if we are able and willing to receive it.

*Dear Jesus,*

*Enable me to suffer the sickness of every child of God, to look beyond my own limitations, and those of the patient's family and caregivers, to bring compassion to the care of these little ones.*

*Help me to care for those who cannot speak for themselves, whose age, disabilities, or illness make verbal communication difficult. Help me to remember that you are the Good Shepherd; you lift these little ones and hold them close to your heart. Help me to employ my heart, as well as my science, to seek out the cause of illness, especially in your smallest sons and daughters. Help me to treat even the most difficult parents with compassion, too. I know it is harder for parents to see their child suffer than to suffer their own illnesses.*

*Remind me that it is a special privilege to help a silent little child back to noisy joy and that witnessing this recovery will be among the greatest rewards of working in the health sciences.*

*In your name,*

*Amen.*

# Fear

*When he saw that they were straining at the oars against an adverse wind, he came towards them early in the morning, walking on the sea. He intended to pass them by. But when they saw him walking on the sea, they thought it was a ghost and cried out; for they all saw him and were terrified. But immediately he spoke to them and said, "Take heart, it is I; do not be afraid."*

*—Mark 6:48-50*

*Peter answered him, "Lord, if it is you, command me to come to you on the water."*

*He said, "Come."*

*So Peter got out of the boat, started walking on the water, and came toward Jesus. But when he noticed the strong wind, he became frightened, and beginning to sink, he cried out, "Lord, save me!"*

*Jesus immediately reached out his hand and caught him, saying to him, "You of little faith, why did you doubt?"*

*When they got into the boat, the wind ceased. And those in the boat worshiped him, saying, "Truly you are the Son of God."*

*—Matthew 14:28-33*

The ambulance was on its way. As I stood plastered against the wall of the ER, rivers of cold sweat ran underneath my shirt. An EMT's voice crackled over the radio, calling out the patient's vitals over and over as the medical staff gathered. Two minutes away. I thought I was going to pass out or throw up. Petrified that I would embarrass myself, I tried to concentrate on the patient, who was at the brink of death.

As part of my pharmacist's training, I was working at a small hospital with a busy ER where pharmacists attended all codes, carrying a black bag full of emergency drugs they could administer as part of the code team. My job as an intern was to observe, answer questions if I could, learn, and stay out of the way.

When the patient was wheeled in, every member of the team swarmed over him, directed by the physician. The man had overdosed; the pharmacist's job was to advise the doctor about drugs needed to detox him or stabilize him, determine doses, and administer them through the direct line the doctor had quickly installed. As I watched the intensive effort to save a patient who had cared so little for himself, my fear was replaced with respect for the staff, admiration for their skills and, finally, great sadness as the color drained from the patient's face and he was pronounced dead, all within a few minutes.

During the month's rotation at that hospital, I attended two other codes, and both patients died. Each time I responded to the code call, as I walked from the pharmacy to the ER, the fear was paralyzing. My head felt frozen, my feelings on fire.

Fear produces clear physiological changes in us when we are in its grip. We first become hyper alert to every detail. Blood pressure rises and blood is channeled to vital organs, muscles to prepare for fight or flight. We sweat profusely, from different sweat glands that advertise our fear. Panic may sweep through us. Our stomachs may churn, refluxing acid. Some people's intestines growl with spasms.

Learning to manage fear is a substantial part of training for health professionals, yet I don't remember talking about it once in school. The first time I viewed a cadaver for study, I was filled with dread. During surgery on lab animals, their chests heaving as they threatened to die even before the awful lab was done, I was fearful. Learning to live with every new fear that surfaced in my training, moving through each stage and managing it, built my ability to help patients manage their own fear.

Patients who are diagnosed with a critical or chronic illness are frequently in a kind of emotional shock, afraid their lives are over. When I realized that I would permanently live with arthritis, it took a long time to accept. I faced my fear by working gradually toward understanding and acceptance.

We all need assistance to overcome fear. As children, our parents secure the closets and look under the bed and pronounce them free of monsters so we can sleep. As adults, we hire lawyers, set aside funds for retirement, and are relieved to get the 'all clear' signal from a good physical. When we are afraid, we are unlikely to make a good decision, weigh alternatives, or have the confidence to try new things.

God does not expect us to manage our fears alone. If we look deep into the scene one night on the Sea of Galilee, we see Peter's wooden fishing boat crashing and rising with the swells, beaten by the wind. From far off, Jesus saw that his disciples needed help and walked out to them, in the midst of the storm.

When the disciples saw him coming, their fear must have exploded. The wind, the raging water, the sweat running into their eyes obscured him, and their fear and imagination twisted his form into a ghost, in their minds. That's when we give up, too. Petrified, we drop the oars and stop trying. Or we scream and panic. That is also precisely when Jesus says, "Don't be afraid! I'm here."

Mark wrote that Peter was the first to reach beyond his fear, saying, "Let me come to you on the water." The gale blowing, the waves looming large, he looked at Jesus and stepped out of the boat. Peter waded toward Jesus a few steps until the fear gripped him again, and he began to sink. This time Peter asked for help: "Save me," he cried, and Jesus did.

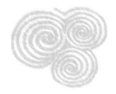

*Jesus will reach to help us,*
*but like Peter we must recognize*
*that we need him and ask his help.*

Jesus will reach to help us, but like Peter we must recognize that we need him and ask his help. No one in the boat that day on Galilee had fallen to his knees and worshipped Jesus when he had fed the five thousand with one small boy's lunch, just hours before. Days of healing the sick, the lame and the blind, fully witnessed by these disciples, had not moved them to shout "Hosanna!" Only when they were gripped with fear of their own, the boat creaking and heaving, filling with water, did they see what he was capable of doing and cry "Save us!"

And of course, the Son of God did.

Dear Jesus,

*I am grateful that you understand fear. You know that fear is a natural response to the threats around us— especially the life-threatening and life-changing illnesses my patients experience. Help me release my own fears to you, reaching to you for strength and courage, so I can be free to respond to them. Help me manage my fear so I am better able to soothe their fears. Help me remember that you know I need you. Thank you that when I call out to you, you will draw near to me, steering me to calmer waters.*

*In your name,*

Amen.

# Burnt Offerings

*"For I desire mercy, not sacrifice, and acknowledgment of God rather than burnt offerings."*

—*Hosea 6:6, NIV*

*Then he went home; and the crowd came together again, so that they could not even eat. When his family heard it, they went out to restrain him, for people were saying, "He has gone out of his mind."*

—*Mark 3:20-21*

Ten years after dropping out of college, I dropped back in—to sixteen solid hours of math and science classes. My chemistry lab section was at seven A.M., and my first task was to light the Bunsen burner. Scraping match after match, the gas hissing away, I could not get a spark. I heard my professor's crisp steps up the aisle. "Can't you light that thing?" he barked, his white lab jacket flapping in my face. Helplessly I shrank back as he grabbed the burner, throttled up the gas, struck a match, and the blue flame leaped up at last.

That harrowing year I learned to set up condensers, flasks and tubes, mastered stoichiometry (the calculated yield from a chemical reaction) and lighting the Bunsen burner on the first try. My teacher was never impressed. While I enjoyed his own "burnt offerings"—demonstrations that might include carving bits of sodium and dropping them into a flask of water, where they would explode in flames—he generally looked down over his half-glasses and stared right through me. Despite the fact that I earned the top grades in his class, after my clumsy failure that first day in lab he had decided I was no chemist. I could never atone for my single failure.

Pharmacy school, the healing science of applying chemistry to the human body, was merciless as well. Expending all of my energy to ultimately help others, I was not very merciful to myself. After I was accepted into professional school, my husband searched for a job nearby, but we reluctantly agreed that only his Portland job would pay enough to support both of us and my college tuition. Away at school, my meals came from the mark-down bin, my winter coat was a raincoat with a flannel lining sewn into it, and my shoes were always soaked through from the cold puddles all over campus. In 1987, the government made no loans to married students who owned even a tiny house like ours, and banks charged eighteen-percent interest. We gave up every cent of extra spending to pay our bills. I drove myself harder and harder, and my husband worked every minute of overtime he could get. We both made huge sacrifices for that degree.

The second year of school was worse than the first. My roommate moved out midyear, and I couldn't afford to keep the rental house we shared, so I searched for the least expensive solo apartment I could find. I accelerated my load to twenty credit hours. Always exhausted, I no longer allowed myself even half a day off each week. In the dead of winter, my car entombed in deep snow, I collapsed next to it one morning in tears with a terrible case of the flu.

School ended in the spring. Now on my feet all day at work, my energy was consumed by my job. Thousands of patients and hundreds of thousands of prescriptions later, I was exhausted. Burning all my free time, I took care of the public during the day, took classes in the evening and volunteered with professional groups with my remaining hours. The intensity of my job hit me one winter, when I worked at a busy pharmacy where the entire staff drank nutritional supplements instead of sitting down for a few minutes to eat solid food. How did this happen?

According to Mark's Gospel, Jesus was once accused of working so hard that it frightened people. The wandering healer and his group had attracted large crowds. One day, so many people jammed into the house where Jesus was that the requests for his help were endless. The man who regarded his downtrodden countrymen as "sheep without a shepherd" could not turn them away. Forgoing food, reaching out to every hand, lifting away paralysis, casting out the evil of illness that appeared to hold each sufferer hostage, Jesus must have worked at a frantic pace.

When his family arrived, distraught and alarmed that his mission seemed to possess him, they tried to pull him away. "He has gone out of his mind!" they cried. Jesus was probably working at a pace that would resemble a bad night at one of our modern emergency rooms. What was alarming to his onlookers at that time has become all too commonplace in modern medical settings, where medical residents work at least eighty hours a week and nurses often work a double shift.

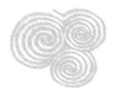

*At the center of intense demand,*
*Jesus had to learn to balance work and rest,*
*just as we need to do.*

At the center of intense demand, Jesus had to learn to balance work and rest, just as we need to do. In later scenes from his years of ministry, he often took time to enjoy dinner invitations from those he met on his travels. When he fed a huge crowd of listeners, dividing bread and fishes abundantly, surely he and the disciples took the opportunity to eat as well. Gospel stories mention occasions when Jesus rested or dozed off and many moments when he simply wandered away in the cool desert evening to be alone with God.

Heading inevitably toward that final altar where his life would be sacrificed for many, Jesus developed a deliberate and masterful approach to time and his limited, human energy. In the many parables he shared with his listeners, it became clear that he, too, learned much from living a fully human life. The lilies growing alongside the road and the small children he scooped up in his arms found their way into metaphors about trusting and loving God. Work, rest and loving the people around him wove seamlessly through his days as he lived ordinary life in an extraordinary way.

Nowhere in the New Testament did Jesus urge his followers to work to the point of exhaustion. Why then do we continue to burn ourselves to ashes on the altar of serving others?

I think back to the time when I watched the staff at that pharmacy down their liquid meals furtively behind the counter. Not long after that, I began re-arranging my priorities. I turned down long Sunday hours, giving myself time to acknowledge the One who provides for my life. Some of the compromises I made, from smaller paychecks to easing out of some volunteer projects, were actually mercies in disguise.

Releasing the control of my time, I let God decide how much I needed to work, I received far more mercy than I had offered myself. No longer sacrificing all my energy on the altar of service, some of my driving ambition burned down to harmless ash.

---

DEAR JESUS,

*You knew what it was to be overwhelmed with people's needs and to live within the confines of a human life. It was not possible for you, in those days before you entered eternal life, to be all things to all people, and it is not possible for me either. It warms my heart to think that you had to learn to balance your giving with your physical energy, just as I must do.*

*Teach me to respect and honor the need for rest and enjoyment that God built into me as part of being human. Remind me when I get overwhelmed that to care for others I need to care for myself.*

*In your name,*

AMEN.

# Sons of Thunder:
# Training and Refereeing Employees

*Jesus went up the mountain and called to him those whom he wanted, and they came to him...Simon (to whom he gave the name Peter); James son of Zebedee and John the brother of James (to whom he gave the name Boanerges, that is, Sons of Thunder)....*

—Mark 3:13, 16, 17

*When it grew late, his disciples came to him and said, "This is a deserted place, and the hour is now very late; send them away so that they may go into the surrounding country and villages and buy something for themselves to eat."*

*But he answered them, "You give them something to eat."*

*They said to him, "Are we to go and buy two hundred denarii worth of bread [eight months' wages], and give it to them to eat?"*

—Mark 6:35-37

"That will never work."
"We've tried that before."
"This place will never change."
Looking around the facility on my first supervisory assignment, I saw a long road ahead of us. The employee roster included those who worked beyond sustainable capacity and others who took two-hour lunches and called in sick a day or two every week. The filing was a mess, seemingly no one answered the phone, and employees were expected to manage themselves. Some employees barely suppressed their hostility toward one another, while others loudly doubted that I had any business trying to fix the hopeless chaos. Yet amongst the storms swirling in that crew, there were bright rays of hope: raw ability, the hard work of many, and hundreds of people who needed our services every day.

One employee stood in the back of the crowd. Petite, blonde, and quite loud, she immediately challenged me: "This place will never change! You're just wasting your time."

As I checked thousands of prescriptions, dug through the files and deflected comments that singed my ego, I remembered John Greenleaf's book *The Servant Leader*, assigned to us by one of my business professors years before. Greenleaf was a Quaker who took the servant aspects of his faith seriously. The opposite of acquisitiveness and power preached in most business texts, servant leadership expands the servant concept Christ lived every day and taught his disciples to practice.

We'd had quite a discussion about the merits of Greenleaf's work during that class. As my professor praised this groundbreaking management approach, my classmate Nancy said, "But this is exactly what mothers have always done!" Others said that to practice real servant leadership in the workplace would be career suicide. How could a servant ever be promoted—or lead, for that matter?

When God called Jesus to start his risky mission, Jesus had no management experience, no formal education in teaching and argumentation, and had never been recognized as a brilliant leader. As a carpenter, he knew that green wood could twist and break as it dried if it was used before it had time to age properly. Though Jesus was green at the task of leadership, there are signs that his human skill and techniques matured as he traveled along in his ministry.

Though Jesus recruited his dozen top people from humble backgrounds—including ordinary fishermen and a government tax collector—they were slow to associate his helping style with their future as leaders in his organization. I can imagine that some evenings, after listening to his disciples bickering, hearing them ask who was the greatest among them, Jesus may well have cried out to God, "How can you expect me to lead this crew?" When his followers squabbled at dinner, Jesus must indeed have wondered, "When will they ever understand me?" Even after Jesus raised the dead and walked across the choppy Sea of Galilee, the disciples still doubted him.

Jesus knew the time was short to train those who would become the foundation of his new movement. Rising to the leadership role, he observed the aptitude of his followers. Simon, whom he renamed Peter (or "the rock," in Greek) and the brothers Zebedee, whom he humorously nicknamed "Sons of Thunder," were privileged to share with him some of the most revealing moments of his ministry.

Jesus never missed an opportunity to teach, even during those months of his final journey to Jerusalem. As he prepared his followers for his inevitable death, warning that he would be leaving them, they still selfishly competed. When James and John demanded recognition and power, Jesus plaintively repeated, "Whoever wishes to become great among you must be your servant" (Matthew 20:26).

Still they failed to understand.

This gentle leader made one more effort to get through to them. Hours before he was arrested, Jesus knelt before them during the Passover meal. Carrying a basin of water, he performed the lowest servant's task in any household: He washed the dusty feet of his friends. Wordlessly, Jesus demonstrated that the greatest must be willing to become the least. Only Peter showed an inkling of understanding of this ritual. At first refusing to be washed by Jesus' hands, in a rush of understanding Peter asked Jesus to wash not only his hands but his feet as well.

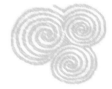

*Throughout his single, magnificent management assignment, Jesus maintained such openness and humility toward his followers that they felt free to voice their every concern to him.*

Though Jesus responded forcefully when the situation demanded, he allowed people to learn at their own pace and searched for multiple ways to demonstrate and teach the principles he wanted to instill. Throughout his single, magnificent management assignment, Jesus maintained such openness and humility toward his followers that they felt free to voice their every concern to him.

Anyone in a leadership role knows what it's like to endure misunderstanding and competitiveness. When I think back to my first supervisory assignment, I think of the high intensity work, usually against the constant backdrop of employee skirmishes. Trying to teach and steer sixty people, I was often approached on my lunch break by someone who wanted to complain about yet another employee. There were constant squabbles, almost always over petty things or home issues that followed someone to work.

After months of backbreaking work, I felt that we had made a bit of headway. As we readied the facility for inspection by one of our national accounts, I heard one of our technicians sitting on the other side of a partition burst forth, saying, "We have to do WHAT? Well, that's *stupid*. We never had to do that before and everything was working just fine."

"I know it sounds stupid," I called from the other side of the wall. "But the inspectors love this kind of stuff, so just do it, okay?"

Five minutes later, I walked over to her side. The tech's eyes were big, and she expected me to be angry. I looked at her and said, "You're a good tech, and you are entitled to your opinion. I respect it. But this time, we're going to do it my way."

We both laughed.

Part of leadership is knowing what our employees really *need* to hear, not what they *want* to hear. Just as suturing a wound is painful and frightening to the patient, some pain may be needed to get any job done. "It hurts," the patient complains. Yet going directly through the hurt is often the best and fastest path to getting better.

Months later, this formerly ragged team received an excellent rating from our national account management team. Every member of the sixty-person crew had contributed good ideas, polished things up, solved problems, and taken pride in their work. I was elated, and so were they.

When these brief moments occur on the job, some would call it a kingdom moment.

DEAR GOD,

*When supervising others, I am sometimes called
to clean up a mess, mediate a conflict between
professionals, kneel on the floor with a roll of duct tape
and do a quick repair job, or listen to the employees sing
the ninety-seventh verse of the "I didn't do it" song.*

*Help me to remember that it's my faith you desire,
not perfect results. I know you love my futile days as
much as my moments of brilliance, and your kingdom
has room for me—and each person I work with—no
matter what.*

*Thank you for the growth and confidence I see building
in each employee and for your gift of grace, which
enhances every job.*

*In Jesus' name,*

AMEN.

# FAITH

# Suffering

*He had no form or majesty that we should look at him,*
*nothing in his appearance that we should desire him.*
*He was despised and rejected by others;*
*a man of suffering and acquainted with infirmity;*
*and as one from whom others hide their faces*
*he was despised, and we held him of no account.*
—*Isaiah 53:2-3*


*"For you always have the poor with you."*
—*Mark 14:7*

Late one rainy afternoon, I looked across the pharmacy counter into the eyes of an old woman wearing a lavender coat a decade out of style. Tucked between two rather loud patients, she looked gaunt and sallow. She told me her purse and medication had been stolen on the bus. She had only two dollars in her pocket and was due for a dose.

Pulling up her computer file, I grabbed the phone to plead with her insurance company, prepared to argue. My patient stood and waited quietly, an undemanding little lavender oasis in the midst of the desert full of cell-phone talking customers. My pharmacy technician raced between the dispensing counter, the cash register, and the other phone, keeping the growing crowd reasonably calm as I waded through recorded options. I finally reached a human being.

When I told the insurance person the woman's story, she said, "There is no provision for lost medication on her plan."

"This woman hasn't got five dollars to her name," I said, irritated. "She will have a seizure and wind up in the ER without her phenytoin. What's that going to do for your bottom line?" There must be only one thing worse than *calling* the help line, I thought to myself, and that would be *answering* the line—all day, every day, listening to pharmacists complain, call after call.

Obvious sighs escaped from some of the customers who were beginning to pile up at the counter, but my patient waited, her hands in the pockets of her polyester coat. No finger tapping, no pacing back and forth. She looked up at me with a hopeful smile.

I heard pages being riffled on the other end of the phone, and finally the voice came back on the line: "Just a moment." My temper was ready to boil over at the delay. I had already decided that I was going to pay for my patient's medicine myself, if it came to that.

The voice came back again, almost whispering: "She can have a once-in-a-lifetime emergency refill."

My surprised, relieved expression startled the little woman in front of me, and her eyes grew big. I hung up the phone, still muttering "once in a lifetime." I turned to catch up the pile of prescriptions on the counter, while my tech re-billed the claim. We gave the lady her bottle of capsules (but not before dispensing one with a cup of water). By that time, everyone else had vanished. She said, "God bless you!" to us, smiled again, and left quietly. My tech grabbed her lunch bag, ninety minutes late, and smiled as she perched on a stool behind a shelf for a quick break. Alone with my thoughts for a moment, I felt strangely light and refreshed.

For days afterward, I thought about this woman and the nature of suffering. Why do some of us suffer so much, while others seemingly do not? Is suffering due to events around us, or does it come from within us?

Faced every day with disease and pain, those of us who provide healthcare are unable to help everyone, but we are bound to try. At closing time in any medical facility, there are always a half-dozen stragglers who walk in at the last minute with needs they characterize as critical. Some of them will have ignored a problem for several days or just let their bottle of pills empty, but others will have a sick child who must be seen or a sick spouse left at home long enough for them to run out and get some badly needed advice.

The deepening health insurance crisis has hit our patients hard, which in turn has changed our own work. Patients are losing medical coverage and are expected to pay more of their own costs—and they are therefore delaying or foregoing seeking care. Healthcare facilities have responded by subtracting staff, lengthening shifts, and increasing the expectations of every employee. The human needs of those who provide healthcare are often last on the list. Feeling ineffective and unable to catch up, our fatigue may block not only the subtle signals of other people's suffering but also our own.

To alleviate patients' suffering, we must first understand our own. I often spend time with the New Testament, studying the change in people who lived and traveled with Jesus. The weekend that Jesus died, the disciples scattered and hid, consumed with their own fear of suffering. Yet several others, including women whom Jesus had healed, followed him to his execution and witnessed his death. At great personal risk, they later returned to his tomb and prepared him for burial.

What had happened to those who followed Jesus to the bitter end of his ministry? What change had they experienced that enabled them to follow when others fled? Did Jesus not only heal their physical or emotional symptoms but also help them resolve their suffering in a radical new way?

Chosen by Jesus to found his church, Peter betrayed him. But Peter was later transformed by Jesus' healing touch of forgiveness after his resurrection. The rest of the disciples underwent dramatic change, too, shedding their fear and suffering to boldly carry the message throughout the region and the world.

Jesus himself had to come to terms with the meaning of suffering. His source of understanding and strength came from knowing that God would provide for him in this earthly life. He followed where he was lead and spent time alone with God every day. Calm and fully alive to every patient, he could clearly see their needs. He was able to bring this serenity to every encounter—even to the final hours of his life.

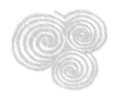

*When we ask God to lead us,*
*God will make use of every experience we have*
*and help us find the best path.*

When we ask God to lead us, God will make use of every experience we have and help us find the best path: We may have to seek more reasonable work hours, if we are overcommitted; we may have to look for new practice settings or completely new ways to employ our skills. Each time we come into God's endless calm, God will help us resolve our suffering, and we will be more able to meet the needs of our patients.

When the woman in the old lavender coat visited me that day in the pharmacy, I saw her as needy and suffering. Instead, she was so patient with me that she let me see how my suffering was preventing me from seeing her clearly. And she taught me this in just a half hour!

Was the old woman really Jesus? Is that why I can never forget her?

---

COMPASSIONATE GOD,

*I ask for your wisdom. Show me how I can help my patients eliminate the causes of suffering that they can change—whether it is securing an egg-crate pad for a bed, making a request for a more realistic job assignment, fine-tuning medication, avoiding dietary choices that cause havoc, or looking for a good support group.*

*Allow my own struggles to help me have compassion for the suffering of others, including my coworkers. Help me to learn from my patients about patience, courage, and keeping a sense of humor about this life. Heal me continually, Gracious God, so I can more completely extend your love to my patients and coworkers.*

*In Jesus' name,*

AMEN.

# Definition of a Miracle

*So they said to him, "What sign are you going to give us then, so that we may see it and believe you?"*

—John 6:30

In the arid heat of the Middle East, ancient hand-written manuscripts were well preserved through the centuries and continue to be found, even today. Scientists analyze every fragment of ancient scripture discovered, and scholars debate its authenticity and evaluate the translations. Books that attempt to prove or disprove the miracles described are hot sellers.

Why do many modern people stumble over the miracles of Christ and endlessly search for proof that they really happened? It's intriguing to consider that what would have been miracles in Jesus' day are commonplace today. Patients who have cataract surgery receive a "second sight." The opening of a patient's clogged arteries gives new life to an old heart. Medications adjust hormones, regulate blood sugar, or cure infections. Healing these ills, in our century, happens every day.

Healing them in 30 A.D., now *that* would have been a miracle.

During the days of Jesus' ministry, there is no doubt that the people crowding around him had cataracts, clogged arteries, imbalances of neurotransmitters, and other illnesses we see today. They also suffered from malnutrition, intestinal parasites, and other diseases that rarely become severe in our modern Western world.

But in 30 A.D. there were no ophthalmologists, no glasses, no corrective surgery, and no eye drops to treat glaucoma. There were no Urgent Care offices, no knee immobilizers, no pharmacies. Jesus may have cleared the cataracts from cloudy lenses, corrected visual focus, or stimulated the sufferer's immune system to overcome a chronic eye infection. When he enabled people to walk, he may have moved stray cartilage from jammed knee joints or freed a nerve that had been entrapped.

Through the arc of time, God has allowed healthcare practitioners to combine generations of knowledge and communicate with one another, enabling us to participate in miracles here and now. We have become so used to miracles that we forget they *are* miracles. For example, researchers long ago discovered the life-saving properties of sterile surgical suites and instruments, which greatly reduced the rate of infection and death of surgical patients. Inventions from refrigeration and freezing to desiccation and aseptic packaging have made it possible to air drop emergency food supplies to isolated refugees, the food appearing on the ground like manna from heaven.

In the 1940s, penicillin was discovered to have bacteria-killing properties. Rushed into development during World War II without time for conventional testing, the drug was administered to soldiers given up for dead. They became walking miracles. In the 1970s, we developed eye drops (and now have their more specific derivatives) that prevented the progression to blindness for a generation of glaucoma patients. In the 1980s and 1990s, we learned to transplant entire organs into dying patients, transferring vital mechanisms of life from a deceased person to enable another to continue to live.

Today's drugs actually assist the body to regain equilibrium by rearranging neurotransmitters (in depression or Parkinson's disease, for example), by relaxing constricted blood vessels, by lowering blood pressure, and by hundreds of other actions. New psychiatric drugs now virtually restore seriously ill patients to normal, clear-headed function, with far fewer physical liabilities than older drugs.

Yet we are still unable to prevent the ravages of Alzheimer's disease, repair the inflamed tissues in Crohn's disease, or enable full recovery from the nerve damage of multiple sclerosis. Curing any of these diseases, which we would consider a miracle today, may be commonplace in thirty or fifty years.

Which is the greatest miracle? That one of Jesus' contemporaries could walk again after he restored a ruined joint two thousand years ago, or that today's surgeon can repair the damage in a few hours in the OR?

Which is the greatest miracle? That Jesus stopped the endless hemorrhage of a poor woman who merely touched him or that today's OB/GYN can accomplish the same miracle with skillful use of medication?

The miracles of Jesus have a timelessness when we consider that some of them now happen regularly. In fact, Jesus said, "The one who believes in me will also do the works that I do and, in fact, will do greater works than these." Perhaps as we produce bio-identical drugs, make cameras that can travel and photograph the digestive tract, and learn how to stimulate brain tissue to eliminate seizures, we are doing the works of Jesus. God has allowed medical science to see and appreciate the design of the human body more distinctly now than two thousand years ago. With that vision comes grave responsibility to use that knowledge to serve God, and thus our patients, faithfully.

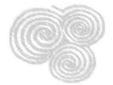

*The true miracle is that we don't always know what the outcomes of our healing efforts will be. Just as our patients do, we must walk in faith, accepting that we participate in a power beyond ourselves.*

Sometimes when I consider the miracles I have seen and in which I have assisted through my professional practice, I am humbled to think that the Master Physician may have first performed them so long ago. Jesus himself may not have been able to explain how he healed those who were psychotic, or epileptic, or burning with raging fever. He reached out in faith, even as today's physicians, nurses, and other healthcare professionals reach out in faith, trusting that God will make the best use of our skills and caring touch.

The true miracle is that we don't always know what the outcomes of our healing efforts will be. Just as our patients do, we must walk in faith, accepting that we participate in a power beyond ourselves. Reaching out to link our hands with God's hands, we translate God's grace through our skills and effort, participating in yet another miracle.

*BELOVED GOD,*

*Rekindle in us our commitment to providing miraculous medical care. Remind us that each patient comes to us in faith, and we will best serve that faith by remembering that the healing arts originated with you.*

*When we begin to take the human body's ability to heal for granted, lead us back to the Master Physician and give us new appreciation for his unlimited faith in you. Though we cannot perfectly heal every patient who presents to us, every patient will notice our caring intentions. Those intentions are the most important link between you, our patients, and ourselves. Let us inspire those we care for to receive the best possible outcome of our skills, contributing their own efforts and faith to the process.*

*In Jesus' name,*

*Amen.*

# Transformation:
## Mary Magdalene's Story

*Soon afterwards he went on through cities and villages, proclaiming and bringing the good news of the kingdom of God. The twelve were with him, as well as some women who had been cured of evil spirits and infirmities: Mary, called Magdalene, from whom seven demons had gone out, and Joanna...and Susanna, and many others.*

*—Luke 8:1-3*

The stories of the New Testament are sparing on details and have been widely interpreted. And women are barely mentioned. This is not surprising, considering that during the historical times of Jesus' life women were regarded almost as property by men. The importance of women in the ministry of Christ must have been quite astounding for them to have been mentioned at all.

Mary Magdalene's life, up to the day Jesus healed her, is sketched in just a few phrases in the book of Luke. In the language of that ancient time, Luke tells us only that Jesus cast out "seven demons" from her. There are numerous clues in the New Testament that what the writers called "demon possession" we would now call epilepsy or mental illness.

In an era when mental illness was regarded as punishment or evidence of sin, Mary Magdalene must have been completely outcast. As a mentally ill woman in a patriarchal society buckling under foreign occupation, her life must have been terrible. If men could divorce their wives over petty matters, it is probable that no one would want to shelter a woman who was not fully in command of her senses.

How did she meet Jesus? Did she just stumble in front of him one day? Did he stumble over her? In the healing stories, Jesus did not knock on doors, searching for the sick. He did not force people to submit to treatment. Perhaps Mary Magdalene made a scene, falling at his feet, too desperate to care if she embarrassed herself or his disciples with her display of need.

One thing we do know: Once Mary found Jesus, she never left him.

Gospel writers mention her more often than any of the other women around Jesus, except for Mary and Martha (Lazarus' sisters) and Jesus' mother, Mary. Mentioned in conflicting, fragmented accounts in the New Testament, Mary Magdalene, Joanna and several others came to Jesus for healing, traveled with him throughout Galilee, and were courageous enough to see his body laid to rest after his death.

What gave these women such courage? Was it gratitude? Or was it more than that? In the dozens of Gospel healing stories, there are few reports of people grateful enough to offer thanksgiving at the temple, and fewer still who searched for Jesus and thanked him. Once their crisis was past, people forgot and went on with their lives. But Mary Magdalene, Joanna, and the other women were different. They not only experienced the life-changing touch of Jesus, but they followed him and contributed their resources.

If gratitude is not enough explanation for this devotion, than maybe the reason Mary Magdalene remained with Jesus is simpler and far deeper: Healing such emotional illness may have taken a long time, even for Jesus. Within every story about Jesus healing emotional illness, I think there is an unspoken moment of silence. I can imagine a person grasping at his sleeve and Jesus directing his attention to the one calling him. Jesus would enter the world of pain and discomfort of this child of God and become fully present to the one who needed him. Maybe the crowd would become hushed. Then, breaking the silence by commanding the evil spirit to leave the one before him, there might have been another moment of complete stillness before Jesus' touch would restore the suffering victim. A moment later, the crowd, shocked to witness the change, might have erupted with noise.

However, there may have been an epilogue, often overlooked or unreported, to many of the healing stories about mental illness. Those who witnessed the event might still have been blind to the dramatic change. Even an individual's own family might have refused to believe the changes they saw. A patient who was outcast might have had no place in society to which he could return. He might not be instantly accepted and believed to be whole by his neighbors. Just as today, the healthy transformation of those who are mentally ill only *begins* with recognition and help from the physician. Those around the patient need to readjust, just as the patient needs to make a courageous effort to find a new place in society, while treatment and counseling continues.

Much of the sheer misery of emotional illness emanates from the ostracism and disenfranchisement experienced by the person who is ill. It is important to note that Jesus did not heal Mary Magdalene and simply send her away. She and several others he healed were drawn to his ministry and were welcomed to remain with him. Did Mary Magdalene first bring other women to him for healing? Was Jesus the focal point of a new community, established for support and continued adjustment to radically new, healed lives?

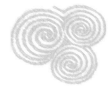

*Jesus not only forgave Mary Magdalene the sins of her life, as he forgives us all, but he also forgave the sins of those who may have caused her pain, whether by wounding her or casting her out.*

Jesus not only forgave Mary Magdalene the sins of her life, as he forgives us all, but he also forgave the sins of those who may have caused her pain, whether by wounding her or casting her out. Mary Magdalene's initial healing continued to be transformed by the richness of this process, yielding the mysterious but powerful outcome of a changed life.

And Mary Magdalene never deserted this true friend, not even at the risk of great peril to herself. In this brilliant and changed atmosphere of living, she was able to rise to her greatest potential, quietly exceeding the devotion of Jesus' closest disciples, who deserted him at his greatest moment of crisis.

Mary Magdalene was rewarded by being chosen to be the first to see Jesus alive Easter morning.

*Dear Forgiving God,*

*Enliven in me your healing power, assisting those
I help to reach their full potential of recovery from
physical and emotional illness. I know that healing
changes may take months or years and may not be fully
appreciated until long after treatment begins. Help me
remember that Christ may have achieved his greatest
healing miracles in those who gave him more than a
few minutes to undo years of suffering and illness and
allowed him to rebuild a healthy person within.*

*Changes within a patient, or within me, may take years
to become apparent to others. The greatest stories of
healing, just as the greatest stories of devotion, may be
told years after I do my part to help someone toward
recovery.*

*In Jesus' name,*

*Amen.*

# Too Late

*When Jesus arrived, he found that Lazarus had already been in the tomb four days. Now Bethany was near Jerusalem, some two miles away, and many of the Jews had come to Martha and Mary to console them about their brother. When Martha heard that Jesus was coming, she went and met him, while Mary stayed at home.*

*Martha said to Jesus, "Lord, if you had been here, my brother would not have died. But even now I know that God will give you whatever you ask of him."*

*—John 11:17-22*

*When Mary came where Jesus was and saw him, she knelt at his feet and said to him, "Lord, if you had been here, my brother would not have died."*

*When Jesus saw her weeping, and the Jews who came with her also weeping, he was greatly disturbed in spirit and deeply moved. He said, "Where have you laid him?"*

*They said to him, "Lord, come and see."*

*Jesus began to weep.*

*So the Jews said, "See how he loved him!"*

*But some of them said, "Could not he who opened the eyes of the blind have kept this man from dying?"*

*—John 11:32-37*

The steepest ascent in any medical career is the divide between life and death.

No matter how well patients are cared for, every patient will eventually die. Every treatment, every drug, every effort to alleviate pain or reknit broken bones or remove suffering reduces to this bare truth: Life is a journey, from birth to death. The job of each healthcare professional is to make that journey as healthy and productive as possible.

Patients may see the view from a different angle. Washed over with information, accustomed to hearing about transplants, incredible life-saving treatments, and miracle drugs, many patients believe that if the emergency room is close enough, the right doctor sees them, or the medevac chopper makes it to the scene in time, everything will turn out all right. The life will be saved, the terrible mistake will be erased, and the accident will not be fatal. Life will go on and death will be defeated.

The more modern medicine offers to patients, the greater their expectations for a good outcome. The greater their expectations, the greater the pressure bearing down on the healthcare provider caught between the patient and death.

Long ago, in a sun-baked ancient land, a human being was given astounding powers of healing. Unschooled and unknown, he traveled on foot from village to village, lifting people out of pain, disability, psychosis, and even death. Without so much as a doorway over which to hang a sign with his name, Jesus welcomed the sick who came to him and sent them home healthy. More than anyone before or since, he translated the touch of God into startling human terms, carrying so much light within himself that disease fled in his brilliant presence.

As stunning as his miracles were, the faith that inspired them was more wonderful still. Calling out in sheer obedience and love, he received power as a sign of the kingdom to come "on earth as it is in heaven," where the restoration of health would be just one dimension of a world realigned with the will of God. In Jesus' humble and complete deference to that kingdom, healing was not the point, just a characteristic of the journey.

Those around Jesus, witnessing his brilliance in pain and need, could not yet grasp the final outcome of a world returned to complete grace. To his followers, Jesus was simply the center, and the healing that came from his hands was an expression of his infallible power.

At Bethany one day, Jesus walked into a scene of misery. His friend Lazarus had died several days before and been laid to rest without Jesus being able to offer even a prayer. Jesus had been close to this family and had stayed at their home several times in those busy years, probably enjoying a welcome retreat, and this particular death filled him with grief.

Both of Lazarus' sisters met Jesus, accusation in their voices, faces contorted with tears, saying, "If you had been here, our brother would not have died." Jesus was filled with his own misery, and the grief of those he cared for deeply cut into him. He broke into tears for his friend, for them, for himself.

The accusation in the sisters' voices really said, "Why didn't you save Lazarus instead of someone else? Why couldn't you save one who loved you?"

In the several days Lazarus had been dead, his body would certainly have decomposed in the desert heat. No one even imagined the possibility that Jesus could call him back to life. But Jesus knew that the still and silent body of Lazarus was a portent of his own coming fate in Jerusalem, where death surely awaited him.

As Jesus approached his friend's grave, struggling to overcome his own emotions and the voices of his enemies muttering in the background, he faced the friends he loved. Enduring their bitterness and extending a loving heart, he healed their faith, and Lazarus walked out of the tomb.

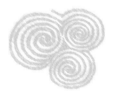

*Enduring their bitterness and extending a loving heart, he healed their faith, and Lazarus walked out of the tomb.*

Of those around him, only Lazarus' sister Mary seemed to grasp that Jesus was preparing to leave them. When Lazarus and his family later hosted a special dinner for Jesus, the Gospel writer John tells us that Mary broke open a jar of burial perfume and poured it over Jesus' feet—a sign that at least one of his followers understood where his life would soon lead.

Across the generations, many healthcare professionals have brought people back from the edge of death. Children are pulled from icy ponds and revived many hours after they seem to die; those who cease breathing, in complete cardiac arrest, resume consciousness; patients whose kidneys stop working, or who have cancer or AIDS or a host of other diseases, now live for years.

Yet no human being will ever again perfectly translate and execute God's caring touch as Jesus did. Human healing will be imperfect. Accusing eyes or voices will cut deeply, tempting even the most selfless to think it's possible to heal perfectly, to understand and do exactly what the patient needs—every time and in every circumstance. But time will run out. Treatments will fail. Patients will die.

Yet we always have the hope and promise implicit in the story of Lazarus, who died and lived again, pointing the way to Jesus' own death and resurrection. When we give our careers to God in faith, we share in a much greater healing mission, knowing that we, too, are moving toward perfect, resurrected life.

DEAR GOD,

*Help us remember that faith, not healing, was the central point of all of Christ's miracles. His life was a living portrait of the coming kingdom, of faith extended to God and the restoration of grace streaming back.*

*In our imperfect world, working with imperfect tools and surrounded by disease, catastrophe and free will, we will never be able to heal everyone or even get to everyone who needs us in time. Remind us that acts of healing toward our patients are our expressions of our faith in you.*

*You will not judge us by the outcomes of our patients' experience, but by the whole-heartedness we extend in helping them. Help us to look and listen beyond the misery of grief and sadness and death in this life, toward what matters most: the coming days of your kingdom, where all will be joined in health and joy.*

*In Jesus' name,*

AMEN.

# What We Have Done
# and What We Have Left Undone

*Then they seized him and led him away, bringing him into the high priest's house. But Peter was following at a distance.*

—Luke 22: 54,

*Then about an hour later still another kept insisting, "Surely this man also was with him; for he is a Galilean."*

*But Peter said, "Man, I do not know what you are talking about!" At that moment, while he was still speaking, the cock crowed. The Lord turned and looked at Peter. Then Peter remembered the word of the Lord, how he had said to him, "Before the cock crows today, you will deny me three times." And he went out and wept bitterly.*

—Luke 22:59-62

Enjoying dynamic lives full of ceaseless action, many Americans regard disease as an annoying interruption. Patients may assume that it's best to *take a pill, have the surgery, get it over with, and move on*. Medical practitioners may respond to this pressure by taking the most aggressive course of action to treat the disease. When treatments fail, however, the lawsuits usually target the professionals, who are accused of doing something wrong: misinterpreting lab tests, confusing medical records, providing the wrong drug or diagnosis.

In medical care, however, what is left *undone* may cost the patient just as much as what is done incorrectly—and it may be much harder to detect. A quick diagnosis and surgery may seem easier than methodical rehabilitation, but it may produce new problems down the road. Failure to permanently change dietary patterns, for example, may do more damage in kidney disease and diabetes than the side effects of medications.

Questions that patients fail to ask may also hurt them. A depressed person may send nonverbal signals to people around him, but if the patient fails to talk about his problem and caregivers hesitate to ask, the illness may prove fatal. Stoics who hide their pain, failing to mention their discomfort to those who could help, may delay treatment for serious illness until they are miserable. The patient who insists on another refill when it is not needed may prevent an essential discussion about long-term side effects.

The night that Jesus' mission came to a horrible end, Peter drew his sword and attempted to protect Jesus from the soldiers who had come to make the arrest. When the other disciples scattered in terror, however, Peter followed, drawn to Jesus by love and loyalty but also fighting his own fears. Courageous enough to be seen, he wasn't brave enough to interrupt the hasty proceedings and save his friend. He failed to act. He remained outside the palace walls and denied knowing Jesus, as Jesus had predicted. When a rooster crowed at dawn, perhaps their eyes met at a distance and broke Peter's heart. He had failed to speak out, to help his friend in great need, and he wept bitterly.

After the resurrection, even Christ's flesh-and-blood appearances to his disciples were not enough to save Peter from his shame. Peter felt as though he alone had failed his friend and driven the nails through his arms. The man Jesus had renamed "the rock," upon whom he predicted he would build his church, was crumbling. Peter needed to know that this failure would not overshadow the rest of his life.

Fishing with his brother a few days later, Peter heard the voice he had been longing to hear. His fragile faith was just strong enough to send him leaping overboard, splashing through the water. In the time it took for the others to haul aboard another miraculous catch, Peter and Jesus were alone for the first time since the resurrection. Perhaps Jesus reached for Peter's hand, to help haul him out of the water, his shoulders heavy with wet clothes and that burden of failure. As Jesus had touched every person he healed, surely the warmth of his hands and his embrace spoke what words can only suggest.

In that poignant scene around a beachside fire, Jesus asked Peter three times if he loved him. Rescued from doubt, Peter was empowered forever to love and follow this friend, who not only resurrected his own life, but Peter's as well.

Working in an imperfect healthcare system, with imperfect skills and tools, there will be crucial questions our patients fail to ask and treatments that will fail to work. We will make wrong decisions. Whether due to our own fatigue, ignorance, or powerlessness, we will not be able to heal every patient.

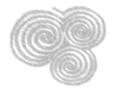

*Only in the endless life of the risen Christ will all of us imperfect, wounded people find perfect healing.*

All of us, healer and patient alike, live and work within a limited life that will end. Only in the endless life of the risen Christ will all of us imperfect, wounded people find perfect healing.

DEAR GOD,

*Caring for patients requires love as well as action. Love for people is the core of healthcare, and following through with each person's true needs is the finest expression of that love through our work.*

*But we are not always able to anticipate every need. We cannot do every task perfectly, every time. Help us to overcome the belief that it all depends on us, that we have complete control over the healing of our patients. Let us remember that only in Jesus' resurrection is found perfect reconciliation, forgiveness and healing.*

*Through the healing miracles of your Son, we see a glimpse of life on earth as you intended it to be. Let us be confident that we can rely on you to assist us in our healing professions. Let us find peace in the example of Christ and his purposeful life. May the Spirit move through us to extend your healing to those in our care. Thy will be done, on earth as it is in heaven.*

*In Jesus' name,*

*Amen.*

# Acknowledgments

Writing a book about healthcare required courage. Writing a book about faith and how it impacts healthcare required inspiration from many people who believe, with me, that God must be in this. Of course, God ever shall be One with every good thing I am able to do.

My husband, Joe, has now survived the publication of my first book and wonders about the other books still in the file cabinet. Thanks for believing in this project and keeping love and dreams alive for thirty years.

Thanks to my editors through the years: my first editor, my mom, who filled our house with books and penciled corrections on my stories; to Harry Cummins, editor of the *Oregon Pharmacist*, who fought the good fight and published only "the good stuff"; to Judy Chi, at Drug Topics, who helped me crystallize a clear, professional voice. Thanks to those at ACTA: editor Marcia Broucek, who knows a good thought when she sees it, asks the right questions, and insists on getting the good stuff on the page; to Greg Pierce, publisher of ACTA, who publishes serious work by women writers—thank you for this opportunity.

Thank you to those who have always encouraged me: Randy Schade; the "three Cheryls"—Cheryll Cormier, Cheryl Worthington and Sheryl Eash Campbell—who read the book and shared their honesty and belief in caring for people; to Sr. Dorothy Pulkka, for spiritual guidance. Thanks to my business professors at George Fox University, Tom Head, Bill Essig (spiritual Godfather), and especially Tom F. Johnson, who has been a great mentor and friend and whose faith helped revive my own.

Thanks to my IT guy, Scott Worthington and his many emergency house calls; to all the great pharmacists I have known and with whom I have worked, who would perish before they would fail to help a patient, especially Cheryll, Randy and Kathy Kelley.

Thank you to the patients I have known through the years and to all those with whom I have worked: physicians, nurses, nurse practitioners, physical therapists, pharmacy technicians and clerks; those who work in the lab, medical records, dietary department, administration, the IT department, and housekeeping; those who make deliveries, process paperwork, drive, or serve as aides. I have learned from all of you. And thanks to the Spirit, which lead me to see something new in those wonderful old healing stories.

# Other Books on Spirituality and Work

*On-the-Job Prayers:*
*101 Reflections and Prayers for Christians in All Occupations*
William David Thompson has put together a series of readings and prayers to be used in the workplace. 128-page, two-color paperback, $9.95

*Spirituality at Work:*
*Ten Ways to Balance Your Life On-the-Job*
Gregory Pierce offers ten "disciplines" that can be practiced in virtually every workplace to raise your awareness of the presence of God and to allow that awareness to change how you do your work. 160-page paperback, $14.95

*How in the World Do We Make a Difference?*
*Getting to the Heart and Soul of Love and Work*
Father Norman Douglas, a Catholic priest, Lawrence Vuillemin, an attorney, and Stephen Hallam, a college professor, combine to take readers on a journey through the struggles we all encounter regarding faith, love and work. 109-page paperback, $9.95

*Holy Vulnerability:*
*A Spiritual Path for Those with Cancer*
Cancer survivor Rev. Donna Schaper outlines eight dimensions of a spiritual path for those with cancer. Blunt, practical, and down-to-earth, she insists on the importance of facing the reality of cancer head on and finding in it a series of unexpected blessings. 92-page paperback, $9.95

*Running into the Arms of God:*
*Stories of Prayer/Prayer as Story*
Father Patrick Hannon, CSC, uses the liturgical hours as a frame on which to hang twenty-one stories of prayer in the ordinary events of daily life. 128-page hardcover, $15.95; paperback, $11.95

*Prayers from Around the World and Across the Ages*
Rev. Victor Parachin has compiled a wealth of sublime, reverent and poignant prayers from many of the world's great spiritual traditions. Each prayer is preceded by a one-paragraph biography of the person who composed it. 160-page paperback, $9.95

**Available from Booksellers or call 800-397-2282**
www.actapublications.com

R. A. Williams Library
Florida Hospital College of Health Science
671 Winyah Drive
Orlando, FL 32803